RECOMMENDATIONS

"This book is an invaluable resource for all those who suffer from CFS/ Fibromyalgia. It provides insight into dealing with the difficulty of performing activities of daily living and serves as inspiration for those who need to realize that they are not alone in their journey."

Kevin V. Hackshaw, M.D.,
Director of Fibromyalgia Specialty Clinics
Program Director, Rheumatology
The Ohio State University
Columbus, Ohio

"By telling the story of her own journey with CFS, Ms. Culbertson has created a handbook that is easy to access while living with this illness. Through her 30 years of personal experience, she offers support and guidance to those most in need."

Cheryl A. Wells, LMT, CHt
Retired NYS Licensed Massage Therapist
Specialized in Medical & Sports
Manhattan, NYC

HELP ME!
What I Wish Families Knew About
ME/CFS

*Myalgic Encephalomyelitis, A Seriously Disturbing Look
At A Seriously Ignored Illness*

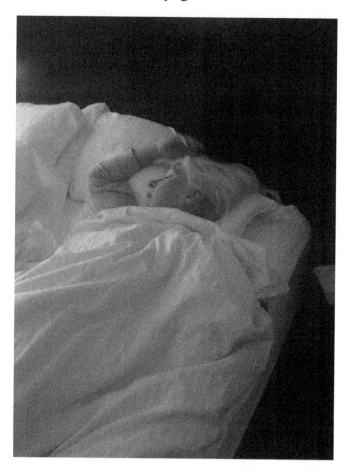

By REBECCA SUSAN CULBERTSON, MSW, LISW-S

HELP ME!

What I Wish Families Knew About ME/CFS

MYALGIC ENCEPHALOMYELITIS (ME)

Also Known As:
CHRONIC FATIGUE SYNDROME

REBECCA SUSAN CULBERTSON, MSW, LISW-S

Copyright © 2020 by Rebecca Susan Culbertson
Print Design by Booknook.biz

Culbertson, Rebecca Susan
HELP ME! What I Wish Families Knew About ME/CFS
Subtitle: MYALGIC ENCEPHALOMYELITIS (ME) Also Known As CHRONIC FATIGUE
SYNDROME (CFS) by Rebecca Susan Culbertson

ISBN 9781654247492
Nonfiction 1. Health and Fitness 2. Diseases 3. Alternative Therapies

This book is dedicated to my husband, Michael, without whom this book would never have been completed, and my life would have lacked a sparkle unlike any other......

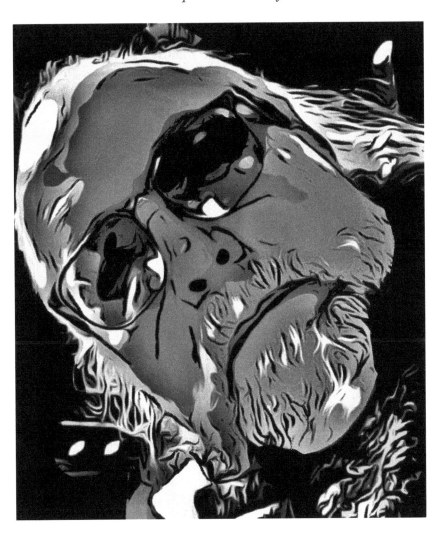

CONTRIBUTORS

Foreword and Therapist Musings
By DR. CHERLA MEISTERMAN, PhD, LISW

Family Support Reflections
By MICHAEL B. MCVICKER, OCPSII

EDITORS

CHERYL A. WELLS, LMT, CHt

MICHAEL B. MCVICKER, OCPSII

DR. CHERLA MEISTERMAN, PhD, LISW

CONTENTS

CHARTING & WORKSHEET INDEX

FOREWORD BY DR. CHERLA
MEISTERMAN, PH.D., LISW

It has been a gift and a privilege to travel beside Susan on her journey to wellness. Susan knew that this illness, Chronic Fatigue Syndrome, required a spiritual and emotional commitment. She had so much to teach us. This is the reason I suggested that she write this book. It required focus, purpose, concentration, and patience. This was an arduous task. We initially set a goal of a few phrases a week on notecards or on the computer. It was important NOT to seek perfection. We had faith that the pieces would come together in time. In one of our sessions we brainstormed about chapter topics and the overall direction of the book. (This is a example of one of the many nontraditional therapeutic interventions that were incorporated.)

Susan requested that I write a chapter from a therapist's perspective. She thought that it may be useful for the individual with Chronic Fatigue Syndrome (CFS) who was unfamiliar with the therapeutic process, and for the therapist who may be hesitant to work with individuals with this illness.*

---

*(Please refer to Chapter 18 to incorporate Dr. Cherla's continuing thoughts for both the CFS patient and the CFS therapist. It is truly teamwork that is necessary in treating this difficult and confusing illness.)

PREFACE

HELP ME! This book pleads for families, partners and friends to educate themselves about this horrific illness that literally rips families apart. Divorce rates are over 75% for couples when a spouse has been diagnosed with ME/CFS. A frightening statistic.

This book is written for those who have been diagnosed with Chronic Fatigue Syndrome (CFS), Myalgic Encephalomyelitis (ME), Fibromyalgia, or any other chronic debilitating disease. It is written for those who are in limbo, suffering still without a diagnosis, and this book is also written to educate families and friends of persons with ME/CFS.

This book will help you learn how to maintain your dignity while dealing with doctors who doubt your illness. You will discover self reporting charts later in this book for use with family, physicians, employers and others. It is difficult to maintain your self confidence if persons in your life do not understand the current state of your functioning. It is of vital importance to educate those around you, when you are able. This book can be a tool to that end.

The book provides information about when and how to apply for disability insurance you certainly deserve. Are you watching your former financial security implode right before your eyes? Learn how to deal with creditors and how to manage financial debt with less stress.

The book will teach you techniques that the author has used in her Family Therapy Practice with patients in living lives of positivity, seeking happiness, and practicing humility. Learn methods of living with ME/CFS while still setting life goals to realistically achieve your dreams.

And importantly, the book is written from the viewpoint of having been diagnosed with ME/CFS herself, and then filtered through her professional perspective as a psychotherapist. Michael McVicker a Prevention Specialist and Family Therapist, concludes this book (in Chapter 26) with THE IMPORTANCE OF HAVING A PERSONAL SUPPORT SYSTEM. Michael uses true life storytelling mixed with humor to inform families from his section titled, A VIEW FROM THE SIDELINE. He tells his story from watching (at times helplessly) and supporting his spouse, the author of this book, through the misery this illness brings. He also writes through the lens of being a stepfather to their two teenage sons, and watching their ascent into adulthood. He deals with topics not currently addressed in other ME/CFS literature currently available, including sex and intimacy. Divorce is seldom the most ecological solution to this real life crisis. Divorce only exacerbates the familial problems.

Dr. Cherla Meisterman, PhD, LISW, (Dr. Cherla's Musings, Chapter 18) offers methods of treating patients with ME/CFS, and attempts to invite other professional therapists to join her in treating this very needy population. With divorce rates so high, questions arise about why more ME/CFS patients do not seek psychotherapy treatment. To me, as a ME/CFS sufferer, it is very clear. Treatment is financially prohibitive, and more importantly persons with this diagnosis have been told verbally and nonverbally, over and over "it's all in your head". So why would any ME/CFS patient *want* to go to psychotherapy? ("Why go and prove the wrong headed physicians correct - "it's all in my head"?) If the patient is supported by his or her partner, and if the patient feels believed that their illness is real, then psychotherapy may become an option that could potentially save relationships and lower divorce rates. Dr. Cherla addresses how to go about selecting the best therapist for you, and things to consider prior to making that phone call.

My hope is this book will serve as a reference, a workbook, a source of sanity, and a small dose of levity for those whom are caught up in this devastating, frustrating illness. So please feel free to cry, laugh, yell, or smile as you explore the following pages. There are worksheets included for your written expression, and for use with physicians, therapists, and other treatment professionals.

Please note, I have often used short sentences to assist the ME/CFS reader with symptoms of brain fog and cognitive impairment. I have also formatted this book into shortened paragraphs, whenever possible to accommodate the reader.

CHAPTER 1

NO SUGAR, PLEASE!

I offer fair warning. I do not sugar-coat my experiences in the following chapters of this book. Myalgic Encephalomyelitis (ME)/Chronic Fatigue Syndrome (CFS) at this stage of medical science is not curable. State of the art protocol is still to treat the symptoms, including any reactive depression that may present as an aftereffect of this illness's dogged persistence and unyielding chronic nature.

ME/CFS may, or may not go into remission. It may, or may not improve slowly over time. It may, or may not respond to various symptomatological treatment regimes. It may, or may not totally incapacitate you. Each person is unique with this illness. Each person responds uniquely to the same or similar medications. But consider that these comments also apply to cancer, heart disease, and nearly all other conditions that do have laboratory diagnostic protocols.

On the other hand, I will also absolutely not exaggerate the bleakness of our situation. There are more and more research projects attempting to find causes, improved methods to diagnose, and treatments than ever before. There are more research funding commitments worldwide, by governments and private entities than ever before.

Part of my own healing and treatment has involved finding the benefits of having had ME/CFS. After many years with a retrospective view, there are situations that were blessed by my seemingly senseless loss of a professional career. Remaining positive and hopeful can help you avoid, or at least lessen a reactive depression that commonly follows months of unrelenting ME/CFS symptoms. I will speak further of this in a later chapter.

It is important not to blame yourself for lack of, or slow improvement. Your ME/CFS body has it's own timing for response to treatment even if the same, exact treatment greatly helped another ME/CFS patient you may know. You may go months or years testing one treatment protocol after another, with no positive response. You may find yourself getting worse with no explainable reason.

It begins to become more clear why doctors are frustrated and annoyed with this illness. They don't know how to "*fix it*", and there is not a simple test to diagnose it. But none of us can give up! New information is being reported and shared in hyper-speed fashion due to the increased global internet linkage of ME/CFS researchers and ME/CFS patients in 2020.

From France to Canada to the United States to the UK, many countries and researchers are working diligently to come up with better answers. Along with the Center for Disease Control (CDC), the Solve ME Website (solveme.org), and the Open Medicine Foundation (omf.ngo) appear to be among the most progressive hope for diagnosis, treatment, research, and political advocacy for this illness. It is important to share information that you discover with your medical team. Patients sharing with caregivers is an important link in unraveling this mysterious illness. Patients sharing with one another can also be an important link, such as passing new diagnostic and treatment information, sharing community resources, plus giving general moral support.

While I suggest there is a responsibility to help others, please know I understand this idea can be overwhelming when you are so very ill yourself. If this is true for you, then this is not your time to help others. *Your responsibility is to help yourself first.*

Most persons improve slowly, some persons go into nearly total remission, some persons have second and third episodes, and a few persons never improve or remit. You must put yourself first until your progress is at a point that you will not do harm to your own recovery by using your strength to help others.

Toward the end of my first episode I formed a self-help group for ME/CFS patients. As a family therapist I took on the role as leader of the group. Even though after most meetings I was exhausted, in hindsight it was a helpful step in my return to part-time work. While it was extremely difficult to leave the group to return to work, I had to put my own health first. I knew I didn't have enough strength and energy to do both. I chose to return to work a few hours a day by using a driver for transportation support, and I sadly gave up my involvement with the group.

Unfortunately, for better or worse, we understand this illness from the inside out. That is the real reason why we must all be there for one another. We understand this illness as no one else can! Even though this illness is devastating to our lives and our professional careers, until there is a cure we must be ready to assist newly diagnosed patients when our strength allows. Until the time that an ecological and efficacious treatment is found, I will continue to seek out and support fellow sufferers plus all our partners in the medical community that recognize Myalgic Encephalomyelitis (ME) / Chronic Fatigue Syndrome (CFS) as a legitimate and real illness!

As you proceed through this book you will encounter differing names for this illness as they were used in my personal diagnoses, during different time periods. For the sake of clarity and to avoid confusion, I will be using the name Myalgic Encephalomyelitis (ME) throughout the latter part of this book. I have lived through so many nomenclatures used to diagnosis this illness over the past thirty plus years, I am confused at times myself in attempting to write about the history and tract of this illness as it moves from one name to another.

CHAPTER 2

30 YEARS AND ONE
GREAT-GRANDCHILD LATER

I could never have imagined that 30 years, four grandchildren and one great-grandchild after first being diagnosed with Epstein-Barr Virus (now ME) in 1987, I would feel compelled to write a book on this topic. That I would feel it necessary to tell my story in an attempt to help others, by trying to push the medical community toward a resolution of diagnosing and treating this illness with the sobriety and respect it deserves.

I believe it is because of the experience of living those 30+ years and fighting this disease with all my being, that I am able, at this point in life to have altered my perception. By setting emotion aside and getting on with the task of exploring and testing theory after theory, I have gained a way of living with Myalgic Encephalomyelitis(ME) that can be achieved by anyone. Anyone, that is, who is willing to persist and stay determined with their day-to-day research. Anyone who can accept setbacks and failure as a given. And, finally, anyone who can recognize success as a gift that will appear in its own good time.

I was trained professionally as a mental health clinician to encounter a problem, research it, study it, and then solve it. The medical and research communities simply ignored information regarding the cluster of symptoms originally coined Epstein-Barr Virus, or more generically, the "yuppie flu" as it appeared to be attacking young professionals at a higher rate than the general population. In 1987 everyone seemed baffled by this disease, myself included. I now think it was because there was no one simple laboratory, radiological, or clinical test to conclusively diagnose this illness. I cringed to think this might be the future of our relationship with viruses.

After I found one group of doctors that had some information and a healthy curiosity, I was evaluated and given several blood titer tests. My results came back with extremely high elevated levels of Epstein-Barr Virus. What I came to discover was that the physicians who actually understood this illness, whatever name it was given, were few and far between. In 30+ years and multiple hospitalizations, I have personally met very few doctors who understand the illness, know how to diagnose it, plus know how to treat it. It is currently treated under several different nomenclatures; Chronic Fatigue Syndrome (CFS), Myalgic Encephalomyelitis(ME), Systemic Exertion Intolerance Disease (SEID), and unfortunately still far too often, depression and/or malingering. New information is continually added to the ME database. The latest research points to the possibility that ME may not always be the result of a virus; that some Myalgic Encephalomyelitis (ME) sufferers do not show any pre-virus causal elements. This again reinforces the idea of *keeping an open mind* until final, definitive research is in.

Thus, my journey began in July 1987 to the current day. Navigating not only the medical system, but other systems I will address later in the book. I will discuss and offer suggestions for dealing with financial systems, government systems, legal systems, insurance systems, and perhaps most difficult of all, family systems.

If any of this sounds familiar, you have probably already lived through your own nightmare scenarios. Do not discredit your own experience as unimportant, worthless, or invalid. For just having made it this far - by searching for a diagnosis, by taking the action of reading this book and other literature, you have begun the process toward equilibrium and regaining control of your life.

The CDC (Center for Disease Control) estimates between 836,000 and 2.5 million Americans have chronic fatigue syndrome or ME. The NIH (National Institute of Health) estimates the number of patients who may be diagnosed with ME or CFS in the U.S. is 1.7 million to 3.38 million. Depending on whose research you read, it is reported there are 17 million to 26 million persons with ME/CFS worldwide.

My greatest encouragement to you as a patient is to trust yourself. You have a **real** medical disease. You are most likely just too tired to educate the entire medical community at large.

Don't despair, we shall do it together. ***One at a time!***

CHAPTER 3

THE MYSTERY BEGINS

June 1983. After having just graduated summa cum laude from the University of Denver with a master's degree in Clinical Social Work, I was elated and ready to conquer the world. I remember an employment section of the Denver Post being passed from one almost graduate to the next during the graduation ceremony, raising the anxiety of one non-employed student to the next. Down the line from row to row, we were in a purgatory of sorts, I suppose. Suspended between living on pennies for six plus years, and the unknown abyss of what's next? I had survived a continual state of study, work, study, test, study, work. I had even survived a bout of Legionnaire's Disease my last semester of graduate school.

I was soon to realize this life experience had been a much easier task than what lay ahead. Keeping up with my sons' ever expanding activities (age 11 and 15 yrs.), paying down a mountain of student debt, and finding employment in a tight job market was my new reality. I was living in the beautiful foothills of Boulder, Colorado, but at that time Boulder had more therapists per square foot than any other city in the country. Being both a pragmatist and a realist, I was compelled to consider alternative living locations. So, after graduation I packed our household treasures and moved back to my mid-western home community to begin the professional phase of my life. I was beyond ready to begin my career and finally have a predictable income. I would be able to provide more for my family, and at the same time have the added pleasure of being able to touch other family's lives. An exciting time of life for me, tempered by my sons' protests of leaving friends and mountain skiing behind!

I settled into our new family nest with my parents, who were delighted to have us back in Ohio. They had made many journeys to visit us and enjoyed their Colorado vacations, but my father was in failing health - a major consideration in my return. Within the first month I began practicing psychotherapy at the local mental health agency, which served six adjoining counties. Being the 'new kid' at the agency, plus the only practitioner of Child and Family Therapy, I was profoundly surprised by the scarcity of resources. The opposite of Boulder's rich depth of available therapists, and multiple lists of competing options. As a result, I found myself with a very full caseload at all six sites.

Local Ohio Mental Health Agency - July 1983

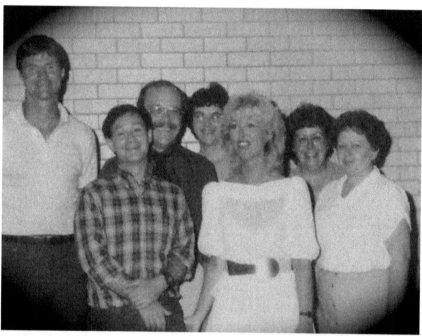

A few of my colleagues in one of the six counties I served. I am in the front row. The director that hired me is on the far left, Mr. Timothy M. Llewellyn. He drove me to all six areas and introduced me to each group of agency staff; the last person I met, on the last day, at the last site of the tour became my husband nine years later.

While this situation was exhilarating with a fertile learning environment, it was also difficult to spend the time I wanted with my sons. My sons attended two different schools, and both had after school sports and programs that pushed the limit for me to arrive on time to their events. Driving to six rural satellite sites - a different county everyday with some day's commuting time adding as much as two hours to an already demanding eight to ten hour workday, was not conducive for a smooth single parent schedule.

The work was rewarding and fulfilling, but the demands of the agency to be a perpetual nomad kept me from feeling professionally grounded to any of the six areas I was serving. I dealt with six juvenile courts, six children's services, six of everything! I was able to keep this pace for over three years, and I learned in depth how different systems worked and how some systems didn't work. However, it eventually became clear this nomadic brand of psychotherapy was never going to allow time for me to pursue my own professional passion and vision, with the depth and control I was ready to build. I knew how I wanted to construct my own practice with the compassion, availability, and environment to nurture my client's healing and growth. It was time for another step forward.

June 1986. With mild trepidation, and wild excitement I resigned from my safe and secure employment. I sought and secured rental of a modest, comfortable office space with an equally modest, and comfortable apartment just upstairs. Travel time had been eliminated and I loved it! I set myself to the task of launching my new private practice. I organized the office policies, procedures, and forms. Happily, I began securing contracts and new patient admissions.

The following picture is of my two sons, Jon and Chad. This was an active and happy time of life for all of us. They were normal teen-agers, but well-behaved, polite and a joy in my life everyday!

Apartment Above Family Therapy Office - October 1986

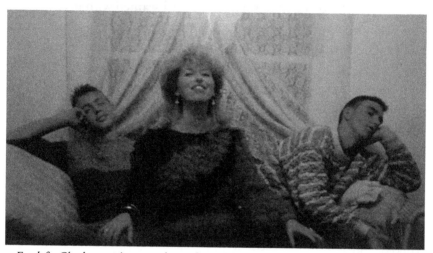

Far left, Chad, age 14 yrs., and Jon, far right, age 17 yrs. This photo was taken just prior to my first episode with ME/CFS. Michael snapped this impromptu photo with the boys pretending to be in a sleep state prior to celebrating my birthday at a "dress up" restaurant. I was in progress of announcing, "Time to go, boys!".
October 1986

My business grew and flourished in the first year. It was more successful than I could have ever hoped or imagined. I had been feeling a little tired, but for good reason. In a little over a year my private practice was bustling. I had a steady clientele, plus multiple school and court contracts. I had tripled my income, and I had just initiated bringing a partner into my practice to help ease the workload. He was also a child and family therapist so I was excited about my successful business endeavor, and the enhanced service we would be able to provide my patients. For the first time, I could plan a vacation without worrying about having enough money and time.

My private life was equally successful. I was happily running to my two teenage sons' school practices and sporting events with my shortened work days, plus I was madly in love. My business partner, Michael, was also my life partner. He brought support not only to my professional life, he brought peace to my soul.

Tri-Valley High School - January 1987

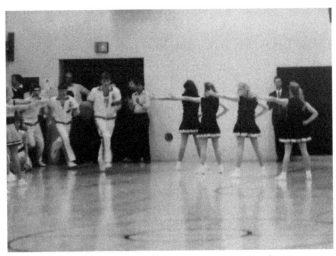

Jon, leading his team onto the floor at a senior year home game.
He played basketball everyday of his life once he began playing. He loved it!

West Muskingum High School - Fall 1988

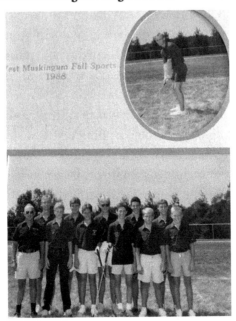

Chad, back row far left, loved playing golf, and remains an avid golfer to this day.
He loved being on teams and was a friend to all!

Michael provided exuberance and fatherly support to my sons. Life was sweet! I decided this was the perfect time for a vacation. So, my partner, my younger son, Chad, and I departed Ohio for the southern shores of New Jersey. My older son, Jon, did not travel on vacation with us this year as he was readying himself for college. (Now ages 15 yrs. and 18 yrs. respectively.)

We headed East toward my sons' favorite vacation spot, Ocean City, NJ; a white sandy beach with a great boardwalk. After a few days at Ocean City, we planned to take our usual route south on the ferry to Delaware and spend a few days at Rehoboth Beach, my favorite vacation spot.

I remember arriving at the ocean breathing in the salty air, and hurriedly unpacking so we could hit the boardwalk. We scoped out the best route from our hotel to the beach, then I reviewed with my son his *do's and don'ts*. We grabbed towels and lotion and headed out. Our first stop on the boardwalk was our favorite cannoli stand, and after a sufficient sampling we were convinced they were as good as the past year's product.

We strolled and sampled treats here and there, and enjoyed the sights, sounds, and smells of the beach. We had a lovely afternoon, a lovely seafood dinner, and then returned to our hotel. We turned in early as we were all a bit tired from the long drive, and our non-stop activity since arrival.

Sunrise the following morning was beautiful, with vibrant oranges and pinks fluttering over the blue lapping ocean waves. We began our day with a relaxing walk on the beach looking for sea shells. We walked leisurely along the shoreline for about a mile, and another mile back to where we began. We did find several perfectly smooth, small shells in lovely neutrals, and a few small pieces of sea sculpted driftwood that would become part of the treasure we would later transport back to Ohio. We ate lunch at a quaint seaside open air restaurant. After lunch, I was ready for a long relaxing soak in the sun.

My madly-in-love partner (now my spouse), who truly *hates* being hot and soaking in the sun, gallantly agreed to sunbathe with me. He carried our beach towels and placed them expertly halfway between the ocean and the boardwalk. It was the perfect spot to sunbathe, while keeping an eye on my nearly 15 yr. old without him suspecting Mother was watching. Chad was happily bobbing in the ocean waves, while we relaxed on the beach. Michael settled on his towel with a book, and I snuggled into my beach towel supported by the warm, white sand. I fondly remember the smell of cocoa butter. Absolute Heaven!

I soaked in the sun for a while, periodically checked on the where-abouts of my son, and began to drift off. Abruptly I sat up realizing I wasn't feeling well. I told Michael I needed to leave. This was **very** unlike me, as I always stayed on the beach until the sunlight waned. I left my towel and my belongings for him to gather, and headed to the boardwalk. In the urgency of those moments, I abandoned Chad with-out informing him of my departure, again, so **very** unlike me.

Confused by what was going on, my partner gathered our belong-ings and Chad, and joined me on the boardwalk. I told him I didn't feel well. I told him I had to get into air conditioning as I couldn't breathe.

I catapulted myself into a boardwalk souvenir shop that had air conditioning. Then my legs gave out, and I was sitting on the floor in the middle of the store. My partner, by now scared and more confused by my behavior said, "What is going on?". I told him I had no idea, but that I needed to get back to the hotel. He called to Chad who had made his way to his favorite arcade, and we all headed back to the hotel. We walked a few steps, sat down on a bench, walked a few more feet, sat down on a bench. Thank goodness we were on a boardwalk that had lots of benches! We walked, sat, walked, sat, walked, ducking in and out of air conditioned shops, until we reached the hotel. A long, slow pro-cess. I stubbornly refused my partner's attempts to call for emergency medical help. After all, we were here on vacation. A vacation that we all had been looking forward to, and I wasn't going to spoil it!

The following day I had recovered a little. I was breathing fine, and was just feeling a little tired. I felt comfortable about not seeking immediate health care. I stayed out of the hot sun, rested and relaxed in the hotel room the remainder of our time at the south shores. It vexed me to not be able to go out into the sun and enjoy the beach as I loved sunbathing, but I decided to relax and just enjoy being on vacation. We stuck to our original travel plans and took the ferry to the Delaware shore, and drove south to Rehoboth Beach for the remainder of our vacation.

At Rehoboth all seemed fine. We cappuccino'ed and shopped (store personnel told me a dress I purchased was identical to one that Kathie Lee had purchased the week before). Upon departure from the dress shop, we further admired my purchase on a nearby park bench as we rested for a while in the shade. I was feeling fine! I decided whatever had happened in New Jersey was over and gone!

The three of us had our picture taken in old time garb for a vacation memory, and then we made dinner reservations at a tiny Italian restaurant highly recommended by the boutique sales staff.

Rehoboth Beach, DE - July 1987

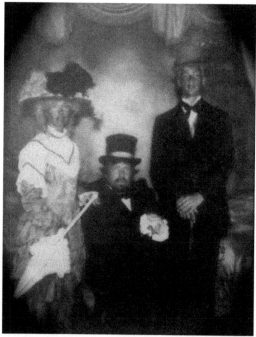

Myself, my partner, Michael, and my son, Chad, just prior to our dinner in Rehoboth Beach a few days after my first onset of ME/CFS symptoms. I was feeling pretty well during the photo shoot, and then later that evening during dinner I experienced another collapse. July 1987

We arrived at the restaurant tanned, relaxed, and ready for pasta. Chad's favorite dish is lasagna, so he was hungrily anticipating this special treat. After we ordered our pasta I decided to allow myself a very seldom enjoyed indulgence of red wine with dinner. We were happy, having fun, and creating family memories. Then halfway through dinner I began to feel ill, and again began experiencing difficulty breathing.

Michael quickly paid for our half-eaten meals, and the three of us departed for the hotel. I felt so bad interrupting our lovely meal, but I didn't have a choice. I certainly didn't want to collapse in public again. We walked slowly with my partner supporting me on one side, and my son supporting me on the other. We paused when necessary for me to rest and catch my breath. Michael was by this time very worried, and Chad was frightened about what was going on with his mother. I was also wondering. What *was* going on?

We headed home the next morning, and I functioned fairly well out of the hot sun. Just riding in the car, I remember being very thankful for the air conditioning. A thought that had never occurred to me on the way *to* our vacation. I had shared driving duties on the way to the Jersey Shore, but driving back home was out of the question. I was uncertain when another episode of exhaustion might strike, or if I might become incapacitated driving through heavy traffic around Washington, D.C. I still was unclear as to when and why these episodes were happening. So I remained a passenger for all our safety, very grateful I had the option for Michael to drive.

My partner wanted me to go see my physician when we returned home, but with the confusing, intermittent symptoms I was hesitant to go. What would I say? When I am in the sun I have difficulty breathing? Or......I had three sips of red wine and I suddenly became weak? From the very beginning of this illness one begins to think of reasons why a doctor might not believe your presenting medical story. With the lack of patient confidence in your own illness, it is easy to imagine why a physician may not be able to grasp the debilitating nature of the symptoms. Especially doctors not yet educated about the mysterious symptoms of what I now know to be Myalgic Encephalomyelitis (ME)/Chronic Fatigue Syndrome (CFS).

CHAPTER 4

SURPRISE DIAGNOSIS

The next day after our return home I resumed my usual work at my beloved private practice, but before day's end I was increasingly tired feeling simply worn out! I noticed I had begun to take a nap around noon instead of having lunch. This was totally out of character for my Type A workaholic personality. Next, I noticed my body didn't want to get up in the mornings. I had to **make** myself get out of bed. My usual habit of jumping out of bed with twenty to-do things in my head had changed to, "Why am I so tired?". My early morning mile long runs which always invigorated me and increased my energy level, had been leaving me fatigued and short of breath. Thus, my previous healthy lifestyle had another inexplicable detriment.

Due to my increasing fatigue and my partner's persistence, I gave in and scheduled an appointment with my local physician. My physician was the spouse of a mental health colleague of mine, so I felt more comfortable approaching them with my strange symptoms than I might have with an unknown physician. I explained my experiences while on vacation, and I gave them a full description of my off and on symptoms of breathing difficulties and fatigue. After a fairly brief physical examination, please try to imagine my surprise when they gave me a diagnosis of depression.

My first reaction was amazement that an educated fully credentialed physician could so clumsily misdiagnose me as clinically depressed. Of course, in my usual therapeutic manner I pointed out immediately that I was actually extremely happy with my current life situation. Madly in love. Operating a successful private practice.

Enjoying parenting two lovely sons. Plus, I had two wonderfully supportive parents. Depression? Really?

I had no history of clinical depression, nor did anyone in my family history. As a therapist, I knew my symptoms did not fit the Diagnostic and Statistical Manual's (DSM)[1] well researched and long standing criteria used to diagnose a person with Clinical Depression. I did know from previous experience within the mental health system, some doctors when faced with the dilemma of not having a definitive laboratory test to diagnose with certainty, will resort to using a psychological diagnosis to explain away the symptoms they are unable to weave into a physical diagnosis.

I informed them my symptoms did not add up to clinical depression. I thought I was giving them an opportunity to self-correct their misdiagnosis, but they steadfastly repeated, "You are depressed". I later realized they simply could not admit the truth. They didn't really know the correct diagnosis for my symptoms. And it was apparent we were not going to change one another's minds. I understood the complex and admittedly confusing symptom presentation they were being confronted with, but making a reflexive diagnosis to soothe their own discomfort is not helpful to the patient!

After departing, my first thought was how very fortunate I had a mental health background with a solid foundation to know this diagnosis was completely wrong. My second thought was, what would other misdiagnosed patients without mental health knowledge do with this sort of diagnosis. Would they believe they were depressed and not seek treatment for their actual illness? I didn't know what illness I did have, but I certainly knew it was **not** a clinical depression.

---

1 *The Diagnostic and Statistical Manual of Mental Disorders provides clear descriptions of mental health diagnostic categories in order to enable clinicians to diagnosis, study and treat various mental disorders.*

CHAPTER 5

THE MYSTERY CONTINUES

The following week Jon and Chad had 4-H projects at our state fair, approximately 60 miles from our home. Michael and I traveled to the fair to support and encourage their efforts in this healthy community activity, and their longterm goal of earning a bit of college money for their futures. Michael enjoyed some fun with Jon and some of his 4-H pals. As we approached the group, our son was engaged in a classic act of late male adolescence. We arrived in the cattle barn just as he was accepting a dare. Jon promptly swallowed a live goldfish freshly retrieved from the midway. The rules apparently included a 10 minute "no barfing" constraint. We later learned he was inspired to this savage accomplishment by the impromptu collection of twenty-five dollars. This was the most radical fair food we encountered all day. Not the type of college fundraising we were expecting, but to this day Jon remains a bold capitalist.

We were having fun and enjoying both boys with their friends. Unfortunately, it was a very hot and humid August day. The light-hearted feeling of being around playful, exuberant adolescents came to a sudden and jarring halt when, as at Ocean City, I couldn't breathe. Again. I was scared, but this time it was accompanied with a splash of anger. I hated worrying my children and my partner with these myste-rious symptoms. All of a sudden I was growing so physically weak I was desperately afraid of collapsing in front of my children.

My partner lead me to the Butter Barn (yes, they carve butter into different sculpture scenes every year, remember this is the mid-west). It was air conditioned to keep the butter stable, and I was hoping it would do the same for me. He propped me up in a chair and left to retrieve the car. Michael arrived at the Butter Barn, and helped me into the air conditioned car. He headed toward help, refusing to hear my pleas of "just take me home" this time.

Michael insisted I see a doctor to ascertain what was wrong, then drove me to the closest hospital which happened to be The Ohio State University Hospital. This is a teaching hospital, and I was assigned to a doctor in residency in the emergency room. After another brief exam, the resident doctor decided I was having a panic attack. My presenting symptoms after exam reflected extremely low blood pressure, slowed heart pulse, labored breathing, and profound fatigue. My limbs felt completely deflated and Michael had to lift me onto and off the exam table.

My symptoms were the complete opposite of a panic attack diagnosis. Michael and I had both treated patients with panic attacks in our professional lives. When the well meaning, inept resident ordered an injection of valium (IM), my partner requested the presence of the supervising doctor. Another doctor quickly arrived at our emergency room cubicle. After looking over my symptoms, the hospital ER physician was baffled and unable to come up with a diagnosis. He did however confirm that it was not a panic attack. The injection order was immediately cancelled. I left the hospital confused and ill without a valid diagnosis. I also left with a hefty bill to pay. I did not have any health insurance since becoming self-employed. I had explored the options of health insurance coverage when first setting up my new office. I researched three different options available to social work clinicians in private practice. The cost of health insurance had been prohibitive. I was a single mother attempting to get a new business off the ground. With a 39 yr. old's fallacy of invincibility, I decided to go without health insurance for a while. Big mistake.

Probably not surprising to many of you, the diagnosis of panic attack remained in my chart at time of discharge. No one bothered to change it.

I returned home exhausted, shaken, and no closer to knowing what was wrong. First I was told I was depressed, now I was told I was having a panic attack. I wanted to find out what *was* wrong, but I was now feeling a little distrustful of the medical community. I didn't want to incur further medical bills if I could avoid it. How could a university teaching hospital so badly misdiagnosis my condition? And then discharge me with an incorrect diagnostic code and no relevant treatment? How could my own local physician misdiagnose me with depression? Was it just me, or was the medical field really this incompetent?

I returned to my regular work schedule and hoped whatever it was, would leave my body, and never return. I was never the one who was sick - I was the one who took care of everyone else!

CHAPTER 6

HOSPITALS, SURGERIES, MEDICAL BILLS! OH, MY!

After returning from our state fair and emergency room excursion, I continued my private practice work, joyously but noticeably still tiring by the afternoon. I did feel relief being back in my familiar surroundings, after living through several scary and confusing episodes. I decided I must have been more tired prior to vacation than I thought. I began working a less hectic schedule to see if I could stabilize my curiously weakened physical state, and to hopefully prevent any more breathing problems. Michael took over the care of some of my current patients, and lightened my workload. Life appeared to be normalizing.

A few weeks later I woke up one morning with a new symptom. It was as alarming and sudden as the onset of my breathing problem at the Jersey Shore. I literally *could not* lift my head off my pillow.

I tried not to panic and scare my son, Chad, and Michael, so I calmly called to my partner and told him I needed help. I told him, "I'm not sure what is wrong, but I can't lift my head." Fortunately he also stayed calm, quickly walked to the side of my bed, cupped his hands under my head, and lifted it up for me. Once I was standing, surprisingly I was able to hold my head upright without any support.

It is no less strange writing this today, than the day it happened. I remember telling my partner and my son, "It feels like a Mack Truck hit me in the back of my head." The back of my head was so sore and sensitive to even the most gentle touch. But no soreness in the front, and no headache! The only other change I began to notice was a feeling of fatigue at the start of the work day, early in the morning instead of the fatigue arriving in the late afternoon.

Somehow I suppressed my reservations, summoned my courage and returned to see my regular physician after the misdiagnosis of depression. I had to find someone or something to help me! I scheduled another appointment, and I could tell they doubted their own diagnosis of depression. I informed them of my recent episodes at the state fair, my experience in the emergency room at OSU Hospital, and my extreme soreness in the back of my head. They decided to refer me back to The Ohio State University Hospital for further research and a definitive diagnosis. They were out of ideas about what was causing the increasing severity of my symptoms, and my decreasing ability to live a normal life.

I arrived back at the university hospital and was admitted as an inpatient. If I had known what was about to happen to me, I would have run screaming into the street and crawled home to my bed. I received twelve days of inpatient testing with a team of eight doctors, and an assorted number of residents depending on the day. By the end of my hospital stay I was totally exhausted, 15 lbs. lighter (a weight loss approximately 15% of my total body weight, at this point weighing 93 lbs.). I had over $40,000 in hospital bills, $10,000 in doctor bills, and every penny to be paid from my depleted self-employed pocketbook, with no insurance, and with still no clear diagnosis. These medical charges were 1987 figures. I wouldn't even want to know the amount of the same charges in today's healthcare market.

The morning of my discharge from this hospitalization I was far weaker. I had to be carried to my bathroom only twelve feet away from my hospital bed. I was too weak to walk a mere twelve feet. I used to relish the exhilaration of hiking in the Rocky Mountains above Boulder, and I always ran at least a mile every morning upon rising. Now I couldn't even make it to my hospital bathroom and back.

While the doctors knew several things I DID NOT have, they had no clear notion of what was causing my many symptoms. I knew with frightening certainty that something was *terribly* wrong. By now I was unable to work, with no health insurance, huge medical bills, credit card collectors getting very nasty on a daily basis, plus I had no idea what was going on with my health. I hadn't applied for disability insurance as I continued to expect I would return to work again soon.

I returned home with a post hospital followup appointment with my regular physician. Due to my complete exhaustion and weakened state, I was now bedfast. Michael was caring for my patients in an attempt to keep my office open, until I could return to work.

I made it to my followup appointment with a great deal of help. Just getting dressed had totally exhausted me. My regular physician conducted a very thorough physical exam, and found a nodule on one side of my thyroid. They said this could explain my fatigue and scheduled me to see a local surgeon immediately. They did not address my other symptoms, other than commenting, "H-m-m, very strange".

I met with the recommended surgeon who ordered not only a scan of my thyroid, but also a mammogram prior to surgery. The mammogram and thyroid scan both showed nodules so instead of one surgery, I was now having two surgeries. In addition, the surgeon informed me he was 99% sure the breast nodule or thyroid nodule was cancerous. He suggested I should make a decision prior to going into surgery whether I preferred a lumpectomy or a mastectomy, if my breast mass was confirmed to be malignant. All I wanted was to go back to my former life - I wanted out of there and back to my practice and my home.

Surgery was scheduled promptly at our local hospital, and I had great hopes that these surgeries would propel me back to wellness. Half of my thyroid was removed, and the nodule in my breast. They were both benign. Great news! I was placed on a medication regime to keep the remaining half of my thyroid active and functioning. I later learned that fibrous masses are common occurrences for persons with ME/CFS.

I thanked my surgeon and left the hospital with a $10,000+ bill. Again, no health insurance. Heavy sigh.

In my weakened post-surgical state, with a negative cancer diagnosis, we began canceling my Family Therapy appointments. I was no longer able to work. I closed my beautiful new office. I was too ill to feel anything except fear. Sadness and anger would hit later.

At the end of both hospital stays I received no indication of what was wrong with me. I did have a lengthy list of what this mysterious illness *wasn't*. Not much help.

This was just the beginning onslaught of doctors, testing, hospitalizations, misdiagnoses, etc. You may be living this scenario yourself. As I later learned, I was not alone. Many other persons with ME/CFS were being diagnosed by the method of symptom exclusion. A common and necessary method, but for me, obviously better in theory than in practice.

OK, now I *was* depressed .... and scared!

CHAPTER 7

RADIO MAGIC

September 1987. After discharge from my last hospitalization, I found myself living in a different home. My partner and my family had not only closed my office and practice, but moved all of our belongings into a house outside the local city limits. I had no income, no child support for my son and no hope of returning to work anytime soon.

Normally, I would have been actively directing *any* change in my life, even a small change! I was so weak from my double surgeries, tethered to my already weakened state, depleted to my core, that I had a passive role in all the changes simultaneously occurring in my life. I was observing through a fog. Somehow I made it from my hospital bed to my family therapy couch in a house foreign to me. I'm sure people were buzzing all around me, taking care of what I could not do myself. I can only now thank them for their kindness from a more distant perspective.

November 1987. I was living a very different life, now acclimating to our new residence, a far more affordable old farmhouse just outside of town, quiet but isolated. My days consisted of lying on our living room sectional couch - the very couch I had purchased for my private practice family therapy room. It was very accommodating for most families with six or seven family members, and larger groups spilled over into accent chairs sprinkled around the room. Now my functional family therapy couch served the purpose of holding my dysfunctional, exhausted body. My bedroom was on the second floor of our new home, which proved too difficult for my shaky legs to navigate without my partner's or son's help. Their work and school responsibilities left me to navigate alone until their return. Our only bathroom was on the first floor. Thus most days I was confined to the ground floor.

I tried to make my bathroom excursions prior to their leaving for work and school. Otherwise, when my legs gave out attempting a solo trip, I would have to finish traveling on hands and knees to and from. It was a huge relief making it back to the couch. My life had so drastically changed. And I didn't know why.

Then, one day, lying on my couch everything changed. Well, not *everything*, but it was a major breakthrough. I was listening to the radio my partner had turned on prior to leaving for work that morning. I was half listening, half listless when I heard a voice begin describing the exact symptoms that I had been experiencing. I sat up and crawled to get a paper and pencil. My hands were shaking while I scratched down his name and the hospital he referenced. The hospital he referenced was in West Virginia. I wouldn't have cared if it was in the Sahara Desert, I would have crawled there on my own if need be. I had found someone who knew what I had!

December 1987. I was able to secure information from the doctor's office of Stephan D. Hanna, M.D., that turned out to be at St. Joseph's Hospital in West Virginia. I phoned immediately. The receptionist said they were being inundated with appointment requests just in the time since the radio program had aired, approximately 30 minutes earlier. She suggested I could make an appointment with a new doctor in their office that had just arrived from The Ohio State University Hospital - such irony! So, I made an appointment with a Dr. Timothy S. Benadum, M.D., who was promised to be supervised by the Epstein-Barr Virus (EBV) expert, Dr. Hanna. Yet to be properly diagnosed, I at least had the name of a syndrome that fit exactly with my symptoms. Finally!!! Progress!!! What I like to call, "Radio Magic".

I will expand on the details later, but after several appointments with Dr. Benadum I was given the diagnosis of Epstein-Barr Virus. It was simple outpatient laboratory blood work at St. Joseph's Hospital that resulted in this diagnosis. It involved a four titer blood test that revealed extremely high Epstein-Barr Virus in my system. Dr. Benadum explained while The Ohio State University Hospital had conducted the same laboratory test with me, they had only ordered a two titer blood work test, but in order to diagnose EBV, a four titer blood test was necessary.

Getting an official *named* diagnosis was at least an emotional relief. At long last I had a *name* for this mysterious illness. This felt like progress even though there were no reliable or proven treatments, protocols, or even an agreement on it's name. What it did do, was validate that I actually had a *real* condition. Now I could move forward to explore new research and potential treatments, while addressing my escalating financial crisis.

CHAPTER 8

APPLYING FOR SOCIAL SECURITY DISABILITY INSURANCE

February 1988. I had always been staunchly independent since I began my first part-time job at age 14 yrs. I began working full time at 17 yrs. of age. I felt very uncomfortable allowing my partner to pay the expenses for my son and me. I flatly refused multiple attempts from my parents to pay our bills. I knew I had to do something to take responsibility to pay for part of our expenses. I bolstered my reserve, armed with my recent diagnosis, and made an appointment with our local Social Security Administration (SSA). I was surprised at how understanding and helpful they were.

They informed me I did qualify to apply for help, *if* I agreed to ask the local court to order child support from my ex-husband. Although this was another stressor, I decided to swallow my pride, go through the unpleasantness of a court hearing, and apply for disability through the SSA. Their main question was "Why did you wait so long to apply?". My answer was simply "Because I kept thinking someone would figure out what was wrong with me, fix it, and I would go back to work!"

Funny how I had always encouraged my patients to apply for help when they were qualified, and needed help. Now I felt it was a weakness to apply myself and admit I needed help, plus admit I was really sick! I had felt independent since I was 14 yrs. old and began my first part-time job. I had always provided for myself, paid my own way to college, and was financially independent. Now I had to admit I needed financial assistance from a source other than myself. I would encourage you to make this adjustment smoother and less stressful than I did. My reluctance only prolonged my pain.

The local Social Security Administration made the process easy, and were graceful in helping me retain my dignity. There were multitudes of papers to fill out. I methodically filled out papers one at a time with the help of my partner. Then, of course, I was denied approval. I cried, then did as the staff at SSA suggested. I had the right to appeal, so I did. I was denied again. I cried. I appealed again, and secured a hearing in front of a federal administrative law judge in our capitol city, Columbus, Ohio. The frustration that you experience in this process is real, but if you remind yourself to just keep moving you will get through it just as I did. Listen to the advice you are given from the SSA staff and then the next step - finding a disability attorney to represent you in your disability hearing.

I discovered one of the most important factors in going in front of a federal judge to request disability insurance is hiring a competent disability attorney who is also respected by the federal courts. You can accomplish this by asking other attorneys and the American Bar Association for their recommendations, and by using a search engine, such as Google for research. Obtain a recommendation specifically for an attorney who is located in the region where your federal court is located. Many judges at every level in the court system are more amenable to local attorneys with whom they are familiar, than they are with attorneys from outside their jurisdiction. Research the percentage of their win/loss cases for your particular disability. Unfortunately, when I applied no one in the State of Ohio had won in federal court for a EBV/ Chronic Fatigue Syndrome disability. The attorney I selected took my case as a professional challenge. I liked him, I think he liked me and I did everything in my power to do exactly as he requested for my case.

Most disability attorneys do not charge any fees upfront, and are only paid if you are approved for disability insurance. Paying for an attorney had been a major concern of mine. I was having difficulty paying my medical bills and credit card debt. How on earth was I going to pay for an attorney? What I discovered, to my great relief, was that I would have to complete volumes of paperwork and assist in preparing my information for my attorney's use in my hearing, but I did not have to worry about paying for an attorney.

The paperwork I collated and assembled is included in the next chapter. My paperwork may not be exact for every organization or agency that you encounter, however, it may be used as a framework you can adjust to meet your needs.

CHAPTER 9

DOCUMENTATION FOR
A SUCCESSFUL HEARING

It is imperative to get information for your hearing collected and collated into a structured format, which will assist your appointed federal judge. My experience revealed that judges and attorneys both need information and education about your life prior to the illness, about the illness itself, how the illness is currently impacting your life, and about the hope you have for your future. *Make it personal, because it is!*

As you begin this most arduous task of collecting information for your hearing in your weakened state, you must ask for help! I couldn't have accomplished all that was needed without my partner; picking up reports, copying papers, composing letters, driving to and from appointments, helping me in and out of vehicles, and handholding!

I quickly learned from my attorney there is no such thing as too much information. As I share the framework for my successful adjudication, you will begin to see the massive amount of documents I submitted with my application request. This was my third attempt at asking for help. I knew for certain I probably was not going to be awarded a fourth!

You do not need to meet with your disability attorney for hours to be more successful in court. Actually, it is the quality of meeting time vs. the quantity which will matter at your actual hearing. Have your questions written down prior to your first meeting, and take a competent advocate with you to record information the attorney recommends you should gather for the court hearing. Remember, with this illness your brain is going to turn to *fuzz* with any amount of stress, and your comprehension is going to be compromised. The amount of physical exertion in just getting to your appointment is going to leave you in a weakened state. I cannot emphasize this enough! Take a family member or friend with you to *all* of your disability hearing appointments. If you find yourself without a support person to assist, it may be helpful to record parts of the meeting with your attorney's permission.

At the very first meeting with my disability attorney, he gave me directions to request my physician attend my disability hearing and present testimony directly to the federal court. Naively, I followed his advice. My physician responded politely, but firmly that he was unable to spend an entire day in court, a fact my attorney apparently already knew. As he had prepared me with the second request. If the physician can not attend a hearing, then ask for a detailed letter. Request that a particular format be used to explain this complicated illness for your court hearing. Have the format readily available to hand to them for their use.

Get prepared to help the professionals you are asking for help. Be as specific as you know how to be when asking busy professional persons for a letter or documentation for a court hearing. While their honest input may be that critical piece that could make a huge difference in your life, it is often an extra chore for them, and an unfamiliar task where clarifying information is genuinely appreciated.

At this first meeting my attorney also gave me a copy of a format for my physician's use, to send information to federal courts for disability determination. My next chore was to take the format from my attorney's letter, and incorporate my personal symptoms and condition in a manner that would assist Dr. Benadum's written report.

I personally delivered a copy of my letter to my physician with a request for written testimony for my disability determination. My physician quickly agreed to the format, and even commented he appreciated a format to follow as a guideline for his letter to the disability court. At the same time I requested all my laboratory reports, all testing and all chart notes from the doctor. He also reported all current research projects and clinical trials in which we were attempting to have me included.

This is a copy of my letter to Dr. Benadum, giving pertinent information that he could use in reporting back to my disability hearing judge in the Federal Courts. This can aide your physician in specifically reporting your symptoms and condition, while making it easier to compose their letter in a shorter amount of time. I have spent much time and space in this chapter on the physician's letter to the federal court, as **this is the most important information the judge will use in their determination of your disability.**

THE LETTER BELOW IS **NOT** A LETTER I USED IN MY COURT HEARING. THIS IS A LETTER I GAVE MY PHYSICIAN TO USE IN WRITING HIS LETTER **FOR** MY COURT HEARING.

Nov. 14, 1988
Dr. Timothy Benadum Xxxxxxx Family Practice 0000 Xxxxxxx
Xxxxxxxxxxx, WV 00000
RE: R.S. Culbertson

Dear Dr. Benadum,
    Thank you for having your office personnel contact me in such a timely manner regarding your decision not to testify in person at my Disability Hearing. I am sorry that you cannot appear in court, but I do understand your hectic schedule demands.
I appreciate your agreeing to write a report using the form letter from my attorney in Columbus. He uses this same format with many physicians in disability cases he is representing.
    (I took a copy of my letter to my regular appointment and gave it to my doctor to secure his agreement to use this particular format, appearing in the Appendix Section at the end of this book. I had previously secured agreement from his office personnel that he would write a disability report for me. I didn't approach his staff about using this format, I waited to make the request in person. It's easier to say 'no' over the phone, so I made the request face-to-face. He actually seemed to like that he had a format to follow. This may not be true of all doctors.)

I suggest the easiest way to organize my information for you would be to follow my attorney's suggested letter structure below. So I will address items in the following order:

*My **symptoms** have been extreme fatigue, general body achiness (muscles and joints), memory loss, inability to concentrate, confused thinking, weakness, dizziness, severe headaches, sore throats, hoarseness, sleep disturbances, mild depression, shortness of breath, bladder problems, sensitivity to light and sound, and with exertion chest pains and irregular heartbeat. These symptoms have persisted since their onset in July 1987.*

*My **test results**: (Please list here.)*

*The Fall of 1987 - Two **surgeries** (Thyroid and Left Breast Lumpectomy) **Medications** Thyroid is regulated with .075 mg. of Synthroid per day. MVP - receiving Persantine 25 mg.*

3 BID, Inderal 20 mg. PRN, and Aspirin 325 mg. per day. Received Elavil now 25 mg. at bedtime for joint aches, mental fogginess, breathing, and sleep disturbances. Motrin 400 mg. 3 BID for joint and body aches. Other empiric trials include vitamin therapy Calcium 200 mg., Vitamin C 500 mg., Vitamin A 5000 I.U., Thiamine (B-1) 1.5 mg., Riboflavin (B-2) 1.7 mg., Niacin 20 mg., Vitamin D 400 I.U., Vitamin E 30 I.U., Vitamin B-6 2 mg., Vitamin B-12 6 mcg., Elemental Iron 66 mg., and Bee Pollen 580 mg. and an exercise program of walking and riding an exercycle without significant or sustained benefits.

Most days I can wash, dress, and prepare meals in microwave; on bad days need help to and from bathroom (stairs) and need to have someone prepare meals; on good days can do light housekeeping and laundry. On a good day can drive self approx. two miles to local mall - need help with grocery shopping as this is still too exhausting. (Even after 12 hrs. of sleep I'm so exhausted it's hard to get out of bed.). Some days I get going by midmorning; other days it's noon or later other days I never do. I have constant fatigue and aching joints.

I will enclose the following information for your use regarding my current situation in which I will cite specific examples:

Employment History

I am a Child and Family Therapist and I used to work 50 to 60 hrs per week in my own private practice. I was also active in my children's school, and managed to run a mile a day in my "spare time". Now I no longer have the stamina to even work. I had to close my office and break contracts that I had already secured. In addition to my private practice I also conducted Trainings and Seminars. I used to lecture "after hours" at local hospitals for their public and in-house educational programs. I have attempted several times to participate in Trainings with my business partner.

He has been willing to do all of the preparation and then to allow me to contribute whatever I can during the actual presentation. My last attempt was Oct. 25 and Oct. 26, 1988. I contributed approximately two hrs. each day, and at the end of the training I had to be carried to the car due to exhaustion and muscle weakness. This was followed by ten days of complete relapse. The first three days I was so fatigued I had to have help to the bathroom, meals prepared for me, and help with personal care. In addition to the exhaustion I had a sore throat, chest pains, palpitations, and my body ached all over. The next seven days I was able to get to the bath and dress by myself, but was so fatigued I had to return to bed the remainder of the day. Even reading was too fatiguing.

Picture Of Life Now

On good days (usually one or two days a week) I can vacuum, do laundry, and drive approximately two miles to our local mall to walk or just sit and "people watch" - these activities are accomplished between periods of rest; and then there are days when I go right back to bed after breakfast. Sometimes reading or talking demands more strength than I have. I can function and "look" almost normal at times, but pushing myself means fatigue, a worsening of other symptoms, and perhaps a week or two of recovery.

Last Spring 1988 I attempted to teach a Psychology Class at a local community college. I taught two classes a week for 1 1/2 hrs. each. I only had to cancel classes twice, but my mother had to come and pick me up approximately half of the time as I didn't have enough energy to drive to class, teach, and then still be able to drive home. I did pretty well the first half of the quarter, but then I began to fall apart the last half. I made it through the week of finals and then was in bed for three weeks following with complete bed rest - my home was a disaster and I had to have help with laundry and cooking. The nice thing that happened from this experience was that I was named Outstanding Part-time Faculty Member for 1988. It allayed some of my worries, as I was afraid I had done a terrible job teaching. I was acutely aware of my limitations, as some days I had to sit down during the entire lecture, and would lose my thought in mid-sentence.

While I have been ill I also have been attempting to write a book (something I have always wanted time to do). Most days I become so frustrated that I can only work on it for approximately fifteen minutes. I used to be a good speller - and now it is a difficult task, having to look words up in the dictionary constantly. I try to read a sentence and I forget what the first half said by the time I get to the end. When I am tired, it is difficult for me to follow conversation - I lose my "train of thought".

I often say things backwards - and repeat things I have said before and don't remember ever saying it. There are times I think my writing isn't making any sense - and I worry when speaking if I am being understood (I was never like this before-communication has always been my strength.) This letter has taken me five attempts to complete.

Since verbal and written work have been frustrating for me, I have also attempted to fill my time with sewing, beadwork and *making jewelry. I can usually work on this for about fifteen minutes before becoming fatigued. On bad days my hands and feet feel like they have weights tied to them, so I'm not able to work on my jewelry, but on fairly good days it helps keep my sanity when I'm too fatigued to get out of bed.*

Chores that required even minimal effort now seem impossible. I vacuum the living room in chunks - I vacuum about a 3' x 3' area, and then rest, vacuum, rest, vacuum, rest, etc.

Lying down is a necessity after even a brief attempt to do anything. I used to clean our entire house and do laundry quickly in my "spare time" from my hectic schedule. Now it's a big deal if I can get the bathroom and kitchen cleaned in the same day or if I can get the entire house picked up and vacuumed in one week; the latter is rare, but a goal I set for myself.

The above information is a description of my general activity and mindset - I'll leave it to your discretion of what to include and how to include it. I have tried to be as accurate and specific as I could be.

One last item before I close, my attorney Mr. Xxxxxx Xxxxxx also advised me that he will need a vitae regarding your Degrees, Licensure, and Speciality Areas, etc.

I lied - one more last item! If you haven't contacted Dr. Xxxxxxxxx yet, I understand that you may want to tape record your conversation with him as he talks incredibly fast and he is difficult to keep up with. Thanks for all your help!

Sincerely,
Rebecca S. Culbertson
CC: Attorney, Mr. XXXXX, Esquire
(1) Enclosure

Please feel free to use my letter as a format for use with your own physician. Replace my information with your own personal information, or reconstruct it to meet your own needs and situation.

Dr. Benadum composed a letter for my use, using the format my attorney gave me. It was tailored to my doctor's medical approach and to my personal medical history. My doctor's letter earned a positive result in my court disability insurance hearing, despite the lack of his physical attendance.

See Dr. Benadum's letter in the Appendix in the back of this book.

Dr. Benadum also included in his packet for the court, thirteen pages of laboratory testing, medication attempts and history of attempts, letters of attempted inclusion into medical research trials with regards to Chronic Fatigue Syndrome and Epstein-Barr Virus, two pages of bio-science laboratory testing for elevated Epstein-Barr Virus serology results utilizing four titers, and three pages of progress notes from my ongoing regular appointments.

My attorney requested that I also gather medical records from all my past physician offices and from the hospitals where I was admitted as an inpatient for testing in 1987, and for my surgeries in 1987. He also had me include records from a previous Transient Ischemic Attack (TIA, Mini-Stroke) in 1984, and records from an episode with Legionnaire's Disease in 1982. He again reminded me that judges need as much information as possible upon which to make their determination.

At this point you may think the document gathering is basically over. But, no. My attorney directed me to obtain written documents about Chronic Fatigue Syndrome/ Epstein-Barr Virus, as it was basically not only a difficult disease for physicians to diagnosis and treat, but virtually an unknown illness to the court system. I found myself heading from one confused system, to another even more confused system, in regards to this disease.

I spent days and nights researching with my partner, and we finally struck gold when we stopped looking at medical research sources, and researched television programming. We heard from a friend who had seen a television interview on *20/20 ABC News titled, "Is That What's Wrong With Me?"*, moderated by Hugh Downs on the evening of July

31st, 1986. It had aired just about one year prior to the onset of my experience with inexplicable symptoms. I phoned ABC News and purchased a written copy of that television interview.

Next I found another television interview from *Lifetime Cable* that aired on August 28th and 29th, 1988, titled *"Chronic Fatigue Syndrome"*. I obtained a copy of their on-air interview and added them to my growing stack of CFS/EBV documentation.

Only in the past few years the evidence of clinically recognized research has proliferated. There are now ongoing research efforts across the globe where the most current information re: ME/CFS is being published and shared You will find many useful resources at the back of this book, in the REFERENCES: RESEARCH section.

SSA Disability Claims *can be* denied due to a lack of information. As I have learned, you will enhance your chance of being approved for benefits by providing as much relevant information as possible.

In total, my attorney gave the federal court judge thirty one exhibits for my hearing. In addition to the previous documents, I also prepared a document with my earnings record showing my progressive increase of income since graduating with my master's degree. I created a document that listed my work activity, i.e., position held with name of employer, job duties and responsibilities, with normal hours worked per week. I included a letter from a local community college, written by the director of their evening programs, where I occasionally taught evening classes in psychology - I requested the director include my teaching skills and work ethic as observed in my quarterly evaluations. I requested a physical capacities evaluation from Dr. Benadum, and a letter from my disability attorney. I also wrote a letter to the judge myself after having it edited by my attorney.

I have spent much time and space in this chapter on the physician's letter. Now, I am going to spend a little more time explaining. Dr. Benadum's letter back to the court reflected much of what I previously sent in my letter to Dr. Benadum, while requesting him to report my information to the court.

See Dr. Benadum's letter to the federal disability court in the Appendix at the back of this book.

My letter to Dr. Benadum was four pages consisting of the following information:

1. My current and past symptoms
2. Past surgeries with dates inclusive
3. Current medications with dosages
4. Past medication trials and results
5. Daily living activities and limitations
     1. What I was able to do professionally before becoming ill
     2. What I could do after Epstein Barr Virus on a daily basis

All of this is in copious detail, as you witness in the preceding letter. Still I want to repeat again this kind of information from your doctor is the most important information your judge will use in their determination of approving your disability, or not approving.

How did I get my doctor to write this kind of information in such a lengthy format? First, I think he believed I was really ill. Second, I think he believed I really wanted to return to work. Thirdly, I provided him with the information that made this kind of letter possible for him to write. You must do the same for your physician.

It is your job to engage your physicians and convince them that their advocacy for your disability hearing is a vital part of your care and active treatment. A physician who is too disconnected, tired, or unconvinced of your need for support beyond the exam room, can most definitely result in doing your treatment and recovery significant harm. I will be discussing in Chapter 21 of this book, what you can do if your doctor is unwilling or unable to assist you in this disability process.

You must make it as easy as possible for your physician to divert from healing time to documentation time. I took that as my responsibility to assist him, so I wasn't in turn causing other patients to suffer from my extra documentation request.

In future chapters, I will be giving you the format I used to document my symptoms and abilities (past & present). Plus, I will be addressing how to change physicians if you are not satisfied with their services, or if you are just not a good fit because of this onerous diagnosis.

You are allowed to have witnesses testify at your hearing. I was the only one testifying in person at my hearing. Your attorney will decide if it is best for you to testify, or not. I would suggest doing as your attorney decides, but I encourage you to ask questions if you disagree with their decision.

The federal judge hearing my case questioned me directly about categories of information that had been submitted in my packet of thirty one entries. He requested I explain to him about my mental impairments, my physical complaints, if I had experienced any lingering side effects from my medications, how often I see my physician, how the Epstein-Barr Virus has affected my daily life, and what a normal day looks like for me now as opposed to my days prior to Epstein-Barr.

Then I was questioned by my own attorney. He asked about my percentage of good days vs. bad days, and the physical difference between the two, about my mental clarity and confusion, and about my physical limitations due to the Epstein Barr Virus.

If you are allowed to give verbal information, my best advice is to paint a picture of what you looked like prior to the illness. Then paint a picture of what your functioning looks like currently, and what symptoms keep you from working. Even if you have a symptom of cognitive disorder (brain fog), do not hesitate to present verbal testimony. If 'brain fog' occurs naturally during your testimony - simply point out the symptom and move on. Do not be embarrassed and try to cover it up. It is part of your current picture. You need to allow it to be viewed by others who are attempting to make a decision in your case.

I also strongly advise taking a family member or close friend with you to advocate on your behalf if you become incapacitated during your testimony. Select carefully. This is a very important part of your recovery. Financial stress can slow your recovery, or propel you backwards into increased fatigue. You need someone that can stay focused with verbal capability, that can speak on your behalf clearly with personal antidotes of your disability. Again, able to explain and describe your before and after functioning.

In conclusion, the steps you need to take to ready yourself for a successful hearing are listed below:

- Research potential disability attorneys
  Date Completed_____

- Recruit friend or family member to be your
  assistant
  Date Completed_____

- Hire and meet with selected disability attorney
  Date Completed_____

- Request information from your doctor's office
  Date Completed_____

- Compose a letter for your doctor with facts
  about how your illness has and is currently
  affecting your life
  Date Completed_____

- Request a personalized letter from your doctor
  Date Completed_____

- Research and obtain educational information
  about your illness to present to your disability
  judge
  Date Completed_____

- Collate and organize all information gathered
  and forward to your attorney
  Date Completed_____

I understand the overwhelming nature of what I have written as necessary tasks for attempting to obtain a positive disability outcome. I suggest chunking it down into small pieces with goal completion dates to help keep you on track. It is so difficult to accomplish anything when you have a chronic debilitating illness. You must remember to ask for help. You can be the organizer of your plan. You do not have to do all the work yourself. Select the time of day when you are at your best, and work in short spurts during that time. If you have increased symptoms on any given day, take the day off. Everyone takes time off when necessary. Don't beat yourself up if you need to take a day off to rest your body and your mind. Just get back to it when you can. Readjust your timeframe as necessary. Keep moving forward. Be kind to yourself!

CHAPTER 10

SUCCESS!!! NOW THE WORK BEGINS!

GOOD NEWS! I received disability based on the illness of Chronic Fatigue Syndrome. My attorney informed me I was the first person in the State of Ohio to receive disability based solely on the symptoms of CFS.

On February 24, 1989, Administrative Law Judge, The Honorable Judge James McElroy issued and signed his Decision on my case. It reads on page 9 of that document:

"Based on the application filed on February 23,1988, the claimant is entitled to a period of disability beginning July 31, 1987, and to disability insurance benefits under sections 216(i) and 223, respectively, of the Social Security Act."

One year from the time I filed for disability it was approved. It lifted a great burden from my shoulders. Now I had enough financial stability to enable me to begin payment arrangements with my creditors. With this relief I proceeded on a path of repayment of medical and credit debt that took the better part of ten years to complete.

The best result of being awarded the official designation of disability was I could focus more fully on my healing. The less than thrilling aspect was having to cope with the label of being a "disabled" person. I certainly wasn't giving up or giving in to this mysterious condition. I was just beginning to fight. Even if it felt at times like I had to fight in slow motion.

(I will speak later in the book about financial issues and how to best deal with creditors, medical and non medical.)

As I focused on my healing, I had several trials of what was considered experimental treatment. For one treatment in particular we traveled from Ohio to Fort Lee, NJ, just outside New York City, for initial acceptance into the program. This treatment did not cure my ME/CFS, but it did help gradually alleviate my symptom of fatigue over a two year period. Keeping current on the latest research papers from any source available to you is vital to your reinstatement of physical health, plus it is a must factor in maintaining the element of hope in your mental health. Many times you learn of new treatments or great doctors from friends and family. I learned about the treatment in New Jersey from a friend in Texas. She was receiving the experimental treatment for her diagnosis of MS and it was helping her greatly. Word of mouth is often the most valuable resource you will find. Do not discount what you can learn from those around you.

With each and every treatment trial, it is extremely important to chart your results on a daily basis. It is important for you to notice and track if a treatment is working, and it is imperative for feedback to your healthcare providers. I always had a PROGRESS SHEET OR A WORKSHEET that tracked my response to different treatments. As I look back, I notice that my worksheets became more sophisticated and detailed as my illness progressed. However, with my initial charting at a time when I could barely walk and mobility limited me to paper and pen, I charted directly onto a calendar.

This is an example of a random week, selected by opening my 1989 calendar to this page by chance. The script is actually what was written on each day. It illustrates the ups and downs of this illness. By transferring this information onto a chart it became a valuable tool to use with my physicians. It helped with knowing when a new medication was indicated, or if a current medication was proving effective or not.

CALENDAR NOTATIONS:
MAY 1989

Friday 12 Chad* Pick up Tux - Get tie for pictures 11-6pm ; Pick up Money - Better day - Couldn't drive, but out of the house, extreme fatigue returned about 3pm.

*Chad - my younger son. Jon -my older son is married & with his wife, expecting child.

Saturday 13 Chad - pictures. Chad - Prom. Return Tie to Hitching Post. 10-4pm. Pick up flowers. Medium day - Drove car into Zanesville. Very shaky in and out. Extreme fatigue about 2pm. Went to mall with Michael about 5pm - had to have help to the car - carried upstairs.

Sunday 14 (Mother's Day)
Bad day. Major aches. Extreme Fatigue all day.

Monday 15 Chad Remainder of money for trip. $90.
Very bad day. Crawled up & down stairs to bathroom. Unable to prepare food in microwave - ate apple. Extreme fatigue, dizzy, aches, heavy chest.

Tuesday 16 Chad Job-Shadowing Atty. Steven Baldwin
Went shopping with Mother. Fair in morning - some tiredness. Extremely fatigued by mid-afternoon.

Wednesday 17 Bad day - in bed all day. Extreme tiredness, heavy chest, difficulty in climbing stairs - was able to microwave food.

Thursday 18 Blank

Friday 19 Bad Day. In bed until evening.

Saturday 20 Chad Dr. Gifford 10:15
Good day. Some achiness.

Sunday 21 Good day! Drove car. Little trouble focusing and concentrating.

Monday 22 Chad $ for trip. $ for contacts.

I shared my calendar notations with my doctor to assist in my treatment. Please note my early charting focused on symptoms and their severity.

The symptoms of ME are many and varied. Thankfully patients do not usually display all of the following list. You may have some symptoms that are constant in your life. Worse some days, better some days. You may exhibit a symptom for a while, and then as it dissipates a different symptom may appear. This is part of the frustration of patients and their physicians as they cope with treating this illness. The chart below may be used to chart and notate your own symptoms. Feel free to cross out the symptoms that do not pertain to you, and add symptoms that are personal to you at the bottom.

Possible Symptoms:

    Persistent fatigue for six months or more
    Swollen lymph glands in neck or armpits
    Sore throat
    Inability to concentrate
    Cognitive disturbance
    Memory Loss
    Muscle pain
    Joint Pain that moves from one joint to another without swelling
    Headaches/Migraines
    Sleep disturbance

Post Exertion Malaise PEM
Non refreshing sleep
Muscular Weakness
Dizziness and lightheadedness

Other Symptoms:

_____

_____

_____

_____

Next, I used a more formal chart, to augment my calendar notations for my doctor's use in treating my ME/CFS during my first episode. It focused completely on current symptoms and their severity. I find it is helpful in notating which symptoms are remitting and new symptoms as they appear. It is not your imagination that symptoms continue to change. That is only partly why this illness is so frustrating and confusing.

You can begin by naming your symptoms to the left on each line. Next you can assign a number to each symptom designating the severity of that symptom. Lastly an indication of whether the symptom is *Steady, Fleeting or Remitting*. Please feel free to change this chart to meet your needs. For example, you may decide to indicate that this is a new symptom previously not charted. This can also be an aide in historical data as to the duration of a symptom and it's response to new treatments.

PROGRESS SHEET: SYMPTOMS OF MYALGIC ENCEPHALOMYELITIS /CHRONIC FATIGUE SYNDROME (ME) / (CFS)

NAME _____

DATE: FROM_____ TO _____

0; 1-mild; 2-moderate; 3-mod. severe; 4-severe

F-leeting; S-teady; R-emitting; _____
Sleep

_____

Activity

_____

Headache

_____

Mental Confusion

_____

Pains

_____

Dizziness

_____

Fatigue

_____

Appetite

_____

Sore Throat

_____

Infection

_____

Muscle Pain

_____

Joint Pain

_____

Fever

_____

Post Exertion Malaise

_____

General Remarks _____

_____

In Chapter 20 you will find a much more advanced charting system I used with my Medical Team during my second episode. During my first episode I focused on symptoms, and as you will read, during my second episode I focused more on activity levels, symptoms and medication trials for charting purposes. I think they both have merit depending on your current situation, and cognitive and physical states. Depending on how much energy you have for charting purposes, may I suggest if your stamina is extremely limited, ask a friend or family member to help you with charting on the days you are unable.

Another use for this charting was to help me realize my personal gains during the long term view of this illness. I never considered obtaining my Social Security Disability Insurance (SSDI) payments as an end into itself. I viewed it as a temporary fix to my short term financial difficulties. I used the victory to allow myself time to recover, so I could one day soon aggressively continue to pursue my career goals. In that moment, however, I was not even thinking of my long term career goals, instead I was focused totally on my recovery!

CHAPTER 11

I'M DOWN, I'M UP, I'M DOWN, I'M UP

Even before you have discovered all the mysteries of this illness, or even before you have a confirmed diagnosis you can begin to tailor your lifestyle to enhance your chance of recovery. Most people do recover from Myalgic Encephalomyelitis (ME) after two or more years, and it is usually a gradual recovery. It is not an illness that you have one day, and the next day it is gone. It is an up & down process with an emphasis on up & down. Research so far shows inconclusive results regarding lifestyle choices, however there are a few known choices that can help.

Exercise at a low level impact can help, but pushing too hard to increase activity intensity, coupled with an increase in difficulty level of exercise ended in a hospitalization for me. I finally realized increasing the incline level on the treadmill, and increasing the speed of my program was agitating my ME/CFS, not helping it. Exercising remains a real dilemma for me. I loved running and fitness training, but now I constantly have to remind myself to curtail my enthusiasm at a level that is beneficial to both cardiac health and ME/CFS health. Slow walking on good days seems to be best for me - and length of walk is much shorter than I like.

Diet is important to even the healthiest of bodies, so of course it makes a huge difference in attempting to reinstate health from the effects of this illness. If you are not sure where to turn with food choices for your health, ask your physician for a referral to a trusted dietitian. Some hospitals offer free classes for the general public taught by their staff dietitians. These are valuable resources that also could help avoid further financial stress, free is always good!

Alcohol and smoking are both contributors to increased symptomatology. It can slow your recovery and increase the severity of your illness. This is the same advice that would be given to an otherwise healthy adult. Excessive use of alcohol and any use of tobacco is detrimental to one's health. It only took a few sips of wine during dinner on my vacation to bring me to the point of needing assistance to walk back to our hotel. Not because of intoxication, but due to the weakening effect it had on my respiratory and muscular system.

Heat and humidity can also increase symptoms of ME/CFS. Finally, the beach, sunbathing, and wine with dinner episodes made sense. This was the explanation for my sudden onset of symptoms during my vacation at Rehoboth Beach. The next step is to take charge, and move on in ways that feel encouraging and supportive to yourself. You can control what you put in your mouth, you can control the type and amount of exercise when you are able to tolerate it, and you can control the temperature and humidity in your daily environment. These are the steps to take charge of your symptoms and head in the direction of recovery.

One of the most debilitating sources that can collapse my energy is mental and emotional stress. Emotional stress is even more devastating to many ME/CFS patients than is physical stress. Emotional stress is immediate and crushing. We know that mental stress, even in small doses, can drain a ME/CFS patient from high energy functioning to a trembly, weak-legged individual in a matter of seconds. The stress of having to deal with medical, or legal, or financial, or any other number of other challenges can kick your overly sensitive flight or fight response into overdrive where you can become physically depleted. This is not an imaginary, "it's all in your head" thing. It is a well researched and documented Mind-Body physical reaction that has been shown to impact us even at the cellular level. If you are interested in the evidence of this, reading Dr. Bruce Lipton's groundbreaking book The Biology of Belief would be a terrific starting point. That is, if you're having a particularly strong and clear minded period when you can focus well enough to read a book at all. The point is this emotional/mental stress is massively REAL; and you will likely encounter many people who will deliver the message that, "it's all in your head" - it ain't. Now for even worse news, emotional will likely be worse (more depleting) than mental stress and the two often show up together and amplify each other. You can be enjoying a fairly normal day, and one stressor that used to be a minor annoyance can flatten the energy and functioning level to becoming bedfast for the remainder of the day, or for multiple days in a row!

Recent (Mind/Body) psychoneuroimmunology findings report how psychological stress manifests itself in the body, and all the more so with a severely compromised immune system. Research in this field can be found at the following website:

https://www.pnirs.org. This can help explain the immediate after-effect of a emotional stress event. Including a psychotherapist into your treatment regime can be another positive link to the restoration of your health.

The following charts may be valuable for you to use as a launching pad to consider the effects of the environment at large on your individual condition.

IDENTIFY FOODS THAT AFFECT YOUR FUNCTIONING

Food Name: (Example: Sugar)	Specify Aftermath Symptom: (Example: Fatigue)
1. _____	1. _____
2. _____	2. _____
3. _____	3. _____
4. _____	4. _____
5. _____	5. _____
6. _____	6. _____
7. _____	7. _____
8. _____	8. _____

IDENTIFY TYPES OF STRESS THAT INTENSIFY YOUR SYMPTOMS

Type of Stress: (Example: Financial Stress)	Specify Aftermath Symptom: (Example: Resulted in 2 Bed Days)
1. _____	1. _____
2. _____	2. _____
3. _____	3. _____
4. _____	4. _____
5. _____	5. _____
6. _____	6. _____
7. _____	7. _____
8. _____	8. _____

By utilizing these additional charts you many be able to discover different patterns of symptom improvement and/or regression. With any chronic illness you need all the advantages you can garner to regain your health, and with ME/CFS your sensitivity to environmental conditions are magnified, and need to be managed with as much precision as your resources and circumstances allow.

CHAPTER 12

FINANCIAL SURVIVAL WHILE DEALING WITH CHRONIC ILLNESS

Many persons who are diagnosed with a chronic illness, whether employed or outside the active workforce are not independently wealthy. Monetary support disruption can lead to extreme stress levels for most of us. The loss of income added to the addition of immense medical costs are common sources of anxiety for the newly chronically ill. 75% of keeping on top of this disease is staying mentally tough. This is a difficult task while in a weakened state of health.

Undoubtably the most consuming stressor connected to a chronic illness like ME/CFS is the financial crisis one may go through. In my situation I delayed applying for any kind of federal or state assistance because I thought I would soon be back to work. Do not do this! Apply for all help possible as soon as possible! All paperwork can be stopped, when your situation improves. Had I applied sooner, I would have had help with all of my costly hospital and doctor bills, which totaled over $60,000. That was in 1980's dollars.

I found myself in the position of being very ill, unemployed, and uninsured. I was self employed and had checked on purchasing health insurance for my family when I opened my private therapy practice. The cost was so prohibitive, I couldn't pay for the insurance and pay rent. Now I had fallen from over $3000 a month income to $0 income. I was in shock, and very ill.

Dealing with financial creditors proactively is the *only* way to cope with the reality of avoiding bankruptcy, and staying solvent through the nightmare that has descended on you. The best advice I can give, and you will find that I repeat this advice often throughout this chapter, is **"Phone them before they phone you"**. Attempt to use the same contact person for ongoing, multiple calls. You should strive to build a relationship and trust with the holder of your credit. Don't make promises you know you can't fulfill. The brutal truth is more difficult to disclose, but failing to keep a financial promise at this point is devastating.

The Health Care System may be aware of their physician's commitment in taking the Hippocratic Oath, but they also become very demanding about payment. I was very distressed about my financial situation as I was used to paying my bills promptly and in full. I explained politely to the medical office that I was still ill and unable to return to work. Their response was to pay my bill with a credit card. I refused, as I knew I couldn't then pay my credit card. I then would receive a lecture about "making larger payments than my current attempts of $2 to $5 a month, or my bill would not be paid off for 604 years". The largest task you have regarding the financial stress is to keep your self esteem intact. To pay what you can each month and **phone them before they phone you.**

I paid $2 to $5 per month on each medical bill. I had been hospitalized three times, I had one emergency room visit, and two inpatient surgeries. I now paid twenty three separate doctor billings, this in addition to regular household bills. I had to close my office after two months of illness because of the enormous overhead without any income. My savings were melting away quickly. You must stay mentally tough to survive!

It is important to ask a trusted family member or friend to assist you with your financial matters, in short, a financial advocate. You can still be in charge of decisions, but there are going to be days when you may be unable cognitively to make sense of financial information. At the very least you may be physically unable to make it to a phone and deal with aggressive collection personnel. Use an answering machine or an answering service. Pass the call information to your financial helper and request that they return the call. Never refuse to respond to a call, no matter how unpleasant. It will only make matters worse. Phone them before they phone you.

A few months after I began contacting my creditors, and I grew more alert and somewhat clearer mentally, I remembered that I had been paying disability insurance on several of my loans and credit cards. I had been sending payments that would have been covered by my disability insurance if I had contacted the companies when I first became ill. Also, I found out the disability insurance policies are not retroactive, so I could not be reimbursed for the payments I had unnecessarily paid since becoming ill.

My second most important advice to a newly chronically ill person, is to have a best friend or close relative sit down with you, and make a list of all your creditors and all your resources, including your bank accounts and income sources. Then request your financial advocate to contact each company. You will need to be in close proximity if you use a financial advocate, to verify authority for your financial advocate to speak "for you". I find a speaker phone works best for this task. Ask your advocate to inquire about disability insurance forms and procedures for temporarily stopping payments. If disability insurance is not covered on your credit cards or car loans, have your advocate request a loan restructure. Most companies are willing to reduce payments if you have a good credit history with them. I found Student Loan payments can be temporarily stopped with a physician's statement as long as you are under the care of a doctor for a recognized disability by the courts.

Important facts for your financial advocate to follow:

1. Make a list of every creditor, medical and non-medical with contact phone numbers, amounts owed, dates of last payment, and proposed repayment schedules.

2. Call each creditor on the list. If you are representing yourself with these contacts, skip to #3. If you have acquired a financial advocate to help, introduce your advocate and announce that you will be on speaker phone during the entire contact period, then move on to #3.

3. Call each creditor on the list - record name of company, date, exact time, contact person's name (ask how to spell name if

needed), why you are calling, and their response - as much in "quotes" as possible.

4. Attempt to contact the same person each time. If not possible, or even if it is the same person, go back to #2 at the beginning of each call. Tell them the date of your previous call, exact time and why you called, and their previous response. Then tell them why you are calling again. Then again follow the same procedure: Record name of company, date, exact time, contact person's name, why you called, and their response.

5. Either have a journal dedicated to your calls, use a spreadsheet, or record information on each bill. Keep bills organized in a folder. You may also use the Financial Contact Log, provided later in this chapter. Use a separate page for each creditor.

6. If you or (your advocate) are not getting the assistance you need from the contact person, if the contact person is rude, or if the financial situation continues to be unsettled, you (or your advocate) should ask to speak to their supervisor. Repeat all of your previous calls with each contact person, giving dates, exact times, and quotes from the contact. You (or your advocate) will be taken more seriously by the supervisor if contacts are documented.

7. If during or following a telephone call, the contact person follows through with a promised action, remember to document their name to use as a future contact person.

FINANCIAL CONTACT LOG*

NAME OF CREDITOR:

_____

_____

_____

_____

_____

_____

_____

_____

_____

_____

_____

_____

_____

*Record: Date, Exact Time, Contact Person's Name, Why Calling, Response of Contact Person in "Quotes"

CHAPTER 13

FUTURE GOALS: DON'T STOP PLANNING

I have always been a planner and methodical thinker. I have always known what my goals were, even when I was still in high school. The only difference in later life is I now write my goals down. I have, since my college days, written down ideas and thoughts, a sort of bucket list. I now write my goals in a more formal manner approximately every six months or so.

About a year after I was diagnosed with Myalgic Encephalomyelitis (ME) I realized I hadn't written down any goals since I became ill. At that point I was freshly diagnosed with an illness I knew nothing about. Would I ever get better? Did anyone ever recover from ME? Would I be like this the rest of my life? Even though I now know the answers to these questions, I didn't at that time.

I just decided to start thinking positive, and I began to set goals for myself, realistic, tiny goals, but goals none the less. Later in this chapter I include a guide to set realistic goals while living with a chronic illness. I set up my goal planner in 1989, not knowing if I would ever be any better physically. Not knowing if I would ever be able to work again. It was a very vulnerable time of life for me. I so very much wanted my professional life back. I knew my next job, if ever able to work again, was going to include healthcare! It was my Goal #1!

The following pages are intended for use in helping you continue to plan your life goals. The important component in this exercise is to set goals as you would have before becoming chronically ill. To adjust to new ways of reaching your goals while realistically coping with ME.

I present this format for your use with any chronic illness goal setting, emphasizing the absolute necessity to adjust your goals to realistic achievement. You are not trying to climb the ladder, or be appointed to the next corporate board. You are trying to regain your footing and balance in life. If you set your initial goals too high, you could be setting yourself up for failure and *extra* stress, defeating the purpose of this mental activity.

As I spent most of my day resting on our living room couch, I often had the thought that I should get up and vacuum the carpet just in that room. Then my mind would remind me that I could barely make it to our bathroom and back to the couch twice a day, sometimes on my hands and knees. I would tell myself I was being silly thinking that I could vacuum that large of a space. I found myself feeling defeated and sad after my internal dialogue, until I decided maybe I should try a small area. So I had my partner set the vacuum where I could access it by the couch before he left for work. He tried to talk me out of it, and looked worried as he departed for work. I smiled an exhausted smile and reassured him it was all fine.

I said to myself, "Let's start with a small plan!" A realistic goal for the day.

CHRONIC ILLNESS FORMULA FOR REALISTIC GOAL SETTING

Date_____

A. Setting mini steps that can be attained, what I name "chunking down" is the first focus of this exercise.

B. The second focus is to never lose sight of your idealized fantasy goals.

    1. Let us begin with a small plan:

        a) Today my goal is_____

        _____

        _____

Small steps to accomplish this are_____

_____

_____

_____

b) By next week I want to have accomplished_____

_____

_____

Small steps to accomplish this are_____

_____

_____

_____

2. Let us move to a larger plan:

a) In six months I will have accomplished_____

_____

_____

Small steps to accomplish this are_____

_____

_____

_____

b)   In one year I will have accomplished_____

_____

_____

Small steps to accomplish this are_____

3.   Let us move to my idealized fantasy goal:

a)   In five years I will have accomplished_____

_____

_____

Small steps to accomplish this are_____

_____

_____

_____

Your goals should be rewritten as many times as you desire. Short term goals can be rewritten weekly or monthly, and long terms goals could be rewritten once or twice a year. You will find that your goals change as your health changes. They may go backwards or forwards, depending on your physical gains or losses. I encourage you to take breaks away from any pressure you may experience if goal setting feels overwhelming at any point. And, you must continue to remind yourself, that is ok! It is more than ok, it is normal for a chronic illness.

Don't forget, be flexible! It is useful to make all of your goals flexible and open to change at any point in time. But don't give up your future goals just because you have been unfortunate enough to have a chronic illness. It should not be an excuse for not achieving. The lack of goals, plus a lack of hope can lead to anger. Anger and frustration can quickly consume the energy otherwise available for goals.

I am extremely happy to report through determination, gains, losses, goal setting and patience, I returned to work in Sept. 1990. I was very shaky, but I planned it as sensibly as I could. I discussed it with my doctor, and we decided that I would start with two days a week, with two days of bed rest in between work days. So, I began working Mondays and Thursdays. We agreed that I would have a driver to drive me to and from work. And if I had a bad day (extreme fatigue), I would adjust the days that I worked that week.

Through my exercise of goal-setting I had secured a part-time contract position that fit my health needs. In Sept. of 1990 I was so excited when I received my first paycheck totaling $320 before taxes. My work report to my local Social Security Administration contained the following remarks: *"I work two days a week, and can vary my hours if I'm not feeling well, and I can change the days I work if I need to health wise. I also ride to work with a co-worker so I don't have to use my energy on driving which helps with my fatigue. I am so excited that I have been able to return to work part-time. I do have flexibility in my schedule - like today I was supposed to work, but I was very fatigued so I will try to work tomorrow instead. I still have fear at times that I will become bed-fast again as the medication I am on is experimental for Chronic Fatigue Syndrome. I would be most appreciative if I could keep my Medicaid for a while as I have no other form of medical coverage. I worry that if I am hospitalized again, before I recover and can afford private health care insurance, I will not have any medical coverage. Thank you in advance for your help."*[2]

---

2 *Dept. of Health and Human Services, Social Security Administration, Form SSA-3945-BK (3-90) Excerpts from Report of Work Activity - Continuing Disability, Submitted by Rebecca Susan Culbertson on March 2, 1991.*

When I returned to full time work and concluded my first journey with Disability Insurance, I wrote a one page *Thank you Letter* to the federal judge that heard my case in court and approved my disability claim. I thanked him for his positive support, and my gratefulness for his determination of disability for Chronic Fatigue Syndrome. I informed him of my return to work, and I encouraged him to consider others who might present themselves in his court with this very confusing illness.

I wanted to encourage this federal judge and the entire disability system to view Chronic Fatigue Syndrome as a credible illness that deserves to be taken seriously; that it is a real threat to a person's health and lifestyle; and that they would consider the next person and all others after me, deserving of disability compensation.

I continue to consider it my duty to educate all persons in this complicated web of illness, as it is intertwined with multiple aspects and systems. It is also my duty to leave a path of kindness to those who help in my recovery, so they are more likely to help others who follow in my footsteps. Kindness and gratitude matter!

Only with great support from my spouse and my family was I able to attempt my goal of returning to work. I cannot emphasize enough the importance of having a supportive network, whether family or friends, in achieving your recovery to health, both physically and mentally. Chapter 26 in this book will expand on this important topic written by my personal support system, my spouse.

CHAPTER 14

WHAT ME/CFS RECOVERY LOOKS LIKE: RETURN TO FULL TIME EMPLOYMENT

During the summer of 1993 I had recovered to the point that I felt strong enough to accept a full time position in administration at a state psychiatric hospital. It had all the characteristics I had charted on my Realistic Goal Setting Chart, achieving full time employment, acquiring medical insurance for myself and my family, 401K potential, professionally challenging, and getting my life back as I knew it.

I accepted the position of assisting in supervision of eight social workers, administrative meeting participation, staying on top of multiple hospital units and nonstop forensic admissions and discharges. I loved it!

At first I had some trepidation about the stability of my health, but after the first month I felt strong and confident that everything was back to normal. I gradually took on added responsibilities through promotions within the state mental health system. In 1998 I moved into an administrative position within the state department itself. I advanced to a governor appointed position, Area Director of Mental Health for Southeastern Ohio. I assumed responsibility for oversight of 20 county community mental health systems, within 7 mental health board areas. I traveled all over the state, and at times assumed national responsibilities with organizations researching mental health issues. I attended state and national conferences.

In April of 2001, I remember one conference in particular. It was a local conference only about one and a half hours from my home. During the last day of the conference, I returned to my hotel room after lunch. I felt very tired, so I laid down on the bed and fell asleep. I never went back to the afternoon sessions. *Very unlike me.* I had a state legislator with whom I was friendly, and planned to visit with her during the afternoon conference. I never saw her, and I left the conference feeling tired and wondering why I hadn't gotten back up to return to my usual networking.

I rested over that weekend, and returned to work the next Monday. I had a huge conference planned for my area of the state, with several mental health and state legislative dignitaries as invited guests. I put the incident behind me and forged ahead with 10 hr. days, planning and preparing for my twenty county area clinical mental health conference.

My normal routine at this time had become, up at 4:30am to make a 1 to 2 hr. commute to that day's work site (within the 20 county catchment territory). Normal working hours were 8 to 9 hours per day with the most forgiving commute, and the return home adding at least another hour or two. My husband reports his memory of my end-of-the-day routine upon arriving home, as eating dinner that he had prepared, and then collapsing into sleep. Our weekends were spent mostly with rest on my part. I loved my job and I was able to keep my hectic schedule under control, with my husband and I both making personal life adjustments. I understood how fortunate I was to have a partner who totally supported my career!

I had had a few incidents of extreme tiredness, and I planned on resting after my major conference was successfully concluded. I had now worked eleven years, slowly, part time at first. But now, I was thriving in my professional position, loving every moment of my work life. I would find a better life/work balance soon.

Columbus, Ohio - March 2001

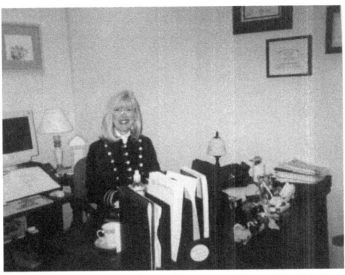

I am working on the Clinical Conference Plans in my office at the Ohio Department of Mental Health. This was approximately three months prior to my sudden second onset of ME/CFS. I remember beginning to have severe headaches at about this time. A totally new symptom absent from my first episode. I had no idea of what was about to happen to me physically.

CHAPTER 15

DEJA VU ALL OVER AGAIN: SECOND EPISODE

My major area-wide clinical conference in May 2001 was a huge success, with all twenty counties in attendance. The conference room was overflowing with talented mental health clinicians eager to share their success stories with one another, with state legislators eager to see how we were spending tax-payer state dollars, and with our state department's Director of Mental Health, Dr. Mike Hogan eager to see how my area of the state was preforming. The most exciting part of the conference for me personally, was watching one of our mental health clients serve as master of ceremonies for the day-long event. And quite successfully serve, I might add!

The conference was held in a lovely historic brick hotel that sits on the banks of the Ohio River. It was a beautiful spring day, and many participants ate their boxed lunches on benches and grasses surrounding the hotel. There were steam wheeler boats and barges passing by that added to the tapestry of spring flowers and chirping birds. We finished the day with a Friday afternoon coffee & tea bar to inspire the final presentations, prior to the usual taxing Appalachian drives home. My husband had attended the conference as a clinician himself, and therefore I had my own personal driver to transport me home after an extremely exhausting week.

On Monday I was back to work, ready to go. This was the budget finalizing time of the fiscal year for all state departments in Ohio. I was consumed with contacting all of my area mental health board directors, and offering assistance to anyone who was panicking or hitting major roadblocks in their own systems.

This went on for two weeks, then on a Friday evening in late May it was dance recital time. Two of my three granddaughters were dancing that night. I loved watching Kelsey and Siena twirl in their sparkly, fluffy costumes! I looked forward to their recitals every year.

I departed from my office 60 minutes away, and I just made the seven o'clock start time in the local community auditorium where they preformed. I was feeling a little tired, but I had the remainder of the weekend to rest and get ready to hit the highway again early Monday morning. The girls both danced beautifully, and I got to bed about midnight.

Saturday morning when I woke, I couldn't get up..... well, not completely accurate. I **could** get up and make it to the bathroom, but the fatigue was so great, I had to immediately return to bed.

I didn't panic. After all, I had all of Saturday and Sunday to rejuvenate before Monday morning. I obviously had just pushed my limits too far by staying up until midnight the evening before. I remained in bed all of Saturday except for 'bladder calls'. My husband fixed meals, served me in bed, and cleared the dishes. I don't remember if I ate anything. I just remember being exhausted; what I now describe as "being tired to my core", a deep internal fatigue.

Upon awakening Sunday morning, the fatigue had not subsided. I barely made it to the bathroom and back to bed. I was so fatigued I was forced to remain in bed again. I was a little worried about my lack of recovery, and was surprised it was going to take another day of rest to get back to my normal activities. I made a mental note to remind myself to slow down when I returned to work on Monday. I knew I was going to have to work fewer hours a day (my usual 10 to 12 hrs., with driving time) so my body could catch up with itself.

Sunday came, and Sunday went.

Monday morning I could not get up. I was **very** worried! I did not want to let my supervisor know how ill I was, nor how frightened. *I did not even allow myself to admit to myself, how ill I might be.* I phoned her and left a message with her assistant that I was taking a sick day, and I would see her on Tuesday. It was unusual for me to even take a sick day. When I had broken my ankle while at work one day, I drove my stick shift car myself to the hospital, and returned to work the following day.

By now you may have guessed, I couldn't get up on Tuesday. I tried and tried. I made it to the living room couch before my legs gave out. I rested a while, but my legs wouldn't support the weight of my body. So I crawled on my hands and knees back to my bedroom. This was such a reminder of my first episode. I had no choice but to admit I was having a ME/CFS relapse. The fatigue was crushing. I was so scared! I had to get back to work! I had bills to pay! I was now buying a home and I had a mortgage to pay!

I loved my job and I had many wonderful projects planned for the spring and summer months. I had so many people depending on me for their jobs to run smoothly, in serving their mental health clients and communities.

I was responsible for all of mental health in Southeastern Ohio. The end of the fiscal year was rapidly approaching. It was imperative that I get back to work. I was responsible geographically for one-quarter of the state. It is the most impoverished area of the state's population; the Appalachian area of Ohio. My area was bordered by Pennsylvania, West Virginia and Kentucky. I felt I was letting people down if I missed even one day of work. I **had** to get my health restored - and quickly!

I gave myself another day to see if I could rebound. On Wednesday morning, I sadly phoned my supervisor, Ms. Judy Wood, LISW, and informed her of my illness, my past diagnosis of CFS and my fears for the future. I sobbed and she comforted me.

She knew my dedication to my work, and to the entire mental health profession. She never questioned my inability to work, or my illness. But she did much more than that for me! She opened the door to a much different experience for my second episode of Myalgic Encephalomyelitis (ME)/Chronic Fatigue Syndrome (CFS).

She quickly explained to me that her daughter, college age, had recently been diagnosed with Chronic Fatigue Syndrome/ Fibromyalgia. Fibromyalgia was a new term to me at that time. When I was originally diagnosed during my first episode, the term Epstein-Barr Virus was used to explain the symptoms. In the eleven years

I had been working again, other patients with symptoms similar to mine were now being diagnosed with Fibromyalgia. Different names, same illness I thought.

I had never been given any information about second or third episodes by any of the medical professionals that had treated me in the past. I guess I had just assumed that once I recovered from this illness, it was gone. After all, I had worked for eleven years after my recovery from CFS!

I knew my supervisor's daughter had been ill, but I knew nothing of her recent diagnosis. Her daughter had gotten married and became ill on her honeymoon cruise. The illness came on so suddenly and fiercely, the cruise ship doctor had her daughter flown by helicopter to the closest land hospital. She was later referred to the Mayo Clinic for testing. I had no idea she had been diagnosed with CFS/Fibromyalgia, and she had no idea I had been diagnosed with the same illness nearly 15 yrs. prior.

My supervisor informed me of a doctor at the local state university teaching hospital (the same hospital that had conducted the intensive, unproductive testing during my first episode), that now specialized in CFS/Fibromyalgia. How uncanny.

Her daughter was a patient of this physician, and she said it was their first hope that maybe someone could help with this strange and unpredictable illness. Her daughter was urgently wanting to get back to her college classes, and had been physically unable to do so since returning from her honeymoon.

She said the doctor was not taking new patients, but she would call and explain my story and see if they would possibly be able to see me for an evaluation. She contacted the specialist's office and secured a referral for me. I was accepted as a new patient. I then phoned the specialist's office and was given an initial appointment date. I was still just as ill as the first episode, but what a difference in the way I was able to handle it. Within six days of realizing the relapse, I knew my diagnosis, and I had found a specialist to treat me. This specialist not only **believed** that CFS/Fibromyalgia was a real illness, but knew the protocol for treatment!

Of course I was in bed most of the time - too fatigued to be normal. But with the support of my husband, I made it to the specialist's office for my first appointment. Even though the doctor had come with the highest recommendation, I found myself doubting how anyone could really do anything about this awful chronic illness.

Could he really get me back to work quickly? Could he relieve the fatigue that was keeping me helpless and dependent on others for daily living tasks? I wanted to work, drive and just be normal again!

This referral was the seed that germinated my idea for having my own personal medical team. I knew this time if I wanted to return to full health, I needed to surround myself with multiple caregivers that could provide answers and assistance that this complicated illness demanded. I wanted professionals that believed this illness was a real thing, that were willing to work together, and pass me from one to the next in a coordinated way that would not exhaust one professional's tolerance and knowledge in dealing with this complicated, complex illness.

CHAPTER 16

MY STRING OF PEARLS: FINDING THAT SPECIAL SPECIALIST

Arriving at my first appointment with the highly recommended specialist, I was both nervous and excited. I walked through the front door and was greeted by a sign that identified my specialist as a rheumatologist. It quickly broadened my world of possibilities. I would never have thought to consult a rheumatologist for my diagnosis of Chronic Fatigue Syndrome. My advice is to remain open to all possibilities and suggestions. You never know where a pearl is going to be hiding, and it's not always in an oyster!

I was pleasantly surprised with the initial paperwork I was given to complete. Of course it had the usual name, address, date of birth, and insurance questions. But then it took a turn into asking relevant questions actually fitting the CFS/Fibromyalgia illness. It was just the first sign that this person may know a little something about my diagnosis, and associated details in living with this illness.

During our initial face-to-face meeting the specialist actually read all of my Intake Questionnaire, listened to my verbal accounts, conducted a thorough physical exam, inclusive of a Fibromyalgia 18 Stress Point Exam, which I had never heard of before. He was able to give me a definite diagnosis of CFS/Fibromyalgia before I left his office. He informed me of the treatment protocol he would suggest, and in detail how he would work with my primary care physician. I hired him on the spot!

Thus began the initiation of my Medical Team Model. It made complete sense to me to have a Specialist treat and help me manage this very confusing and difficult illness. And, it made complete sense to have a Primary Care Physician (PCP) manage my general overall health and normal annual testing (i.e., mammograms, pap smears, bone scans, etc.).

My Specialist's protocol included sending a follow-up letter to my PCP after every visit at his office, with a request for my PCP to forward a copy of my regular laboratory test results to his office to avoid duplication of services. Now it was up to me, the patient, to assist in making this a working model between my Primary Care Physician (PCP) and my CFS Specialist.

My PCP initially verbalized an agreement to receive followup letters from my CFS Specialist, and to forward my laboratory tests to the specialist's office. However, after months of slow improvement and several acute episodes, it became clear that my PCP was Myalgic Encephalomyelitis (ME)/Chronic Fatigue Syndrome (CFS) weary. I learned I had to take responsibility for keeping my Medical Team connected and interested in working together on this complicated diagnosis. It was clear things were going to fall apart if I didn't take charge. So, I secured a new PCP, and fired my current primary care doctor. A sample of the structure I used to hire and fire is found in Chapter 22 of this book: The Eight Step Guide For Changing Doctors.

My new PCP was familiar with ME/CFS, and had other patients diagnosed with ME/CFS. She was pleased and seemed relieved that I was seeing a Specialist, and had no problem with sharing my laboratory test results from her office. She was, in turn, appreciative of the specialist being willing to send her an update of my condition after every appointment with him. I finally had my first two pearls in place!

At this point my Medical Team Model looked like this:

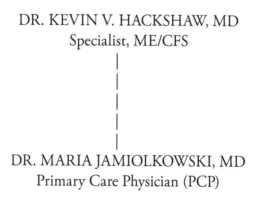

DR. KEVIN V. HACKSHAW, MD
Specialist, ME/CFS

DR. MARIA JAMIOLKOWSKI, MD
Primary Care Physician (PCP)

All laboratory reports flowed into Dr. Hackshaw's office from Dr. Jamiolkowski's office, and all patient visits with ME/CFS treatment recommendations and medication trials flowed from Dr. Hackshaw's office back into Dr. Jamiolkowski's office. I rarely discussed any ME/CFS issues with my PCP. She instead attended to my cholesterol levels, bone density, and occasional influenzas. I sought my ME/CFS treatment from Dr. Hackshaw, and accordingly reserved my ME/CFS questions and new research finds for my appointments with him.

CHAPTER 17

MY GROWING STRING OF PEARLS

I worked in the private sector prior to my first Myalgic Encephalomyelitis (ME)/Chronic Fatigue Syndrome (CFS) episode , thus I received my disability income through the Social Security System. This time I had not even had time to consider disability income as I was once again determined I would return to work asap! I was currently using my sick leave and now my vacation leave time to get by.

During one of many phone conversations with my administrative supervisor, now my guardian angel, she informed me that my sick leave hours were almost exhausted. We then discussed the subject of my co-workers offering to gift me some of their sick leave hours to help out until I filed for disability leave. They requested to remain anonymous, thus I have never had the opportunity to thank them for their generosity. They will never know how very much it meant to me.

She then announced that I needed to apply for disability leave through the state system in the very near future. My immediate thought was, "Oh, no I don't! I'm going back to work!" After reality set in, my second thought was, "Oh, no! Another system to learn to navigate!"

Interestingly, the state system proved to be less paperwork than the federal system, but the medical testing remained consistent. The doctor that saw me for my disability approval, told my husband and I during my examination that he didn't believe in ME/CFS. But he signed my disability papers as an accommodation to my referring doctor. ME/CFS as a diagnosis remained under the care of psychiatrists, with a prescription to treat depression. I was highly insulted *both* times. I swallowed my anger and my pride, as the alternative of no income and certain bankruptcy was not really a viable choice. This time the state system required that I hire a psychiatrist to oversee my care, and to prepare a written report back to them once a year. I continue to challenge the medical system to recognize ME as the physical illness that it certainly is.

Since my profession was in the mental healthcare field, I arranged to see a Dr. Meisterman, who practiced in a city outside my professional geographical area. I decided it would be too awkward to ask a professional in my supervisory area to provide my treatment. I didn't want to make anyone uncomfortable, and I thought it would be unethical and a conflict of interest for me to employ their services, as I had previously had oversight of their agencies in my state department position.

After using my screening protocol for interviewing a potential new doctor, I was delighted to add Dr. Meisterman to my string of pearls. She was well aware of the ME/CFS diagnosis, and had treated other patients in her private practice. She was not only willing, but extremely eager to co-ordinate my care with Dr. Hackshaw. She agreed to completing paperwork required by the state disability system.

I received a letter from the state disability system informing me that my doctor, Dr. Meisterman, did not have the needed credentials to complete my required paperwork. I should have known, everything was going too smoothly! She had a PhD, and I needed an M.D. to meet the paperwork requirements. Dr. Meisterman referred me to one of her colleagues, Dr. Jenkins, M.D., with highest recommendation.

I subsequently met with Dr. Jenkins, and found my fourth pearl. She also had treated other persons with ME/CFS, and was curious and interested in current research regarding this diagnosis. She spoke of treating a reactive depression as a secondary result of this horrific illness, not as a primary diagnosis of a clinical depression. Progress! She also requested that I continue to see Dr. Meisterman for talk therapy and for assistance in completing the required state disability paperwork.

The connection between these two doctors ended up being a blessing, and has aided greatly in my up-and-down, and sometimes sideways, recovery. They were both extremely supportive of my treatment with Dr. Hackshaw, and completed my Medical Team Model.

MEDICAL TEAM MODEL

DR. KEVIN HACKSHAW, MD
Specialist, ME/CFS

DR. CONNIE JENKINS, MD — — — — DR. CHERLA MEISTERMAN, PhD
Psychiatrist, ME/CFS   Psychologist, ME/CFS

DR. ISMET OZKAZANC, MD[3]
Primary Care Physician

---

3 *I was forced to change PCP's due to insurance reasons, not medical care issues.*

CHAPTER 18

DR. CHERLA'S THERAPIST MUSINGS

[This chapter is written by Dr. Cherla Meisterman to inform the reader of how a Talk Therapy Session could enhance treatment of ME/CFS, and also to provide a framework for a therapist who may be interested in working with CFS patients. Reminder: This is one therapist's method of treatment, and other methods may be just as therapeutic with different patients. Therapy is definitely not a one size fits all, but this is presented as one possible model.]

Susan requested that I write a chapter from a therapist's perspective. She thought that it may be useful for the individual with Chronic Fatigue Syndrome (CFS) who was unfamiliar with the therapeutic process, and for the therapist who may be hesitant to work with individuals with the illness. As a therapist you have a right to responsibly refer a consumer on if a chronic illness, such as Chronic Fatigue Syndrome is not an area you wish to treat. It is not my intent to present therapeutic jargon, research, or didactic information.

If you are contemplating entering the therapeutic process, try to talk to the therapist on the phone prior to the first appointment. I recommend that you have a list of questions prepared, such as: what has been your experience working with people with chronic illness, what is your approach in treatment, tell me what the first appointment might be like, etc. As a consumer of behavioral health, you have the right to select a therapist that is a good match, given the confines of your insurance plan or what you can financially afford. It is ok to ask for help in assessing if your insurance will pay for your treatment.

The therapeutic relationship is the main avenue to healing. If you are uncomfortable with what you hear, keep looking until you find someone with whom you feel comfortable. Consider the background of the individual. Do you prefer a therapist that can work with your family? You may have the option of choosing between a psychologist, social worker, marriage and family therapist, or counselor. Since I am licensed as a psychologist and as an independent social worker, my bias is that each discipline has excellent practitioners. I recommend working with someone who is licensed in their field with at least three years of experience. Word of mouth is one of the best guides to finding a good psychotherapist, or you may ask your doctor for a referral.

I am not an expert in dealing with CFS or fibromyalgia. The people with the illness are the experts. They are my teachers. I hold up a lamp so that they can see their way. I have attended my share of workshops, have a background in the health care field, and consider myself a generic practitioner. The way I conduct treatment is always unique to the individual, with certain central beliefs. I will respect the individual's process, I will provide a safe environment, I will offer interventions that are appropriate to the individual, I will not harm the individual in any way and I will abide by the ethics of my professions. I never believe that my way is the right or the only way to healing. It is simply the path that I follow, with the help of God. I know that it is bold for a therapist to mention God. I warn clients that spirituality (not religiosity) is intertwined in my work and if they are uncomfortable with the inclusion, I am not the best choice for them. Susan was accepting, on this condition.

There are a few concessions that I make with individuals who carry this diagnosis. I do not charge for missed appointments as long as a call has been made to cancel. My usual policy requires 24 advanced notice. There have been numerous times that Susan has been unable to attend appointments without the advanced notice due to the unpredictability of the illness. On one occasion, she was driving to the appointment and was too weak to continue driving. I do not need to add to her stress by adhering to strict financial rules. (This is the luxury of being a partner who is in private practice.) I call my CFS clients prior to their appointments, if I have a cold and give them the option of rescheduling. I do not want my health to tax their immune system.

I believe that bodywork is an important adjunct to talking therapy with CFS clients. Pain is a typical symptom and physical relief is mentally calming. I encourage appropriate referrals to manage pain. We must remember some people are uncomfortable with touch, and that is to be respected. Susan's husband received Reiki Training to aid Susan and himself.

Since Susan has beautifully described the issues we addressed, I will focus on the interventions. Our priority was relieving symptoms of depression, due to the second reappearance of CFS and loss of her professional self. We examined Susan's diet, exercise, milieu at home, relationships, and fears for the future. We began with the most tangible, diet. Susan chose to eliminate sugar, eating small meals throughout the day, including as many organic food sources as possible. She incorporated brain booster foods, such as foods rich in omega threes, and vegetables with vibrant color to boost her immune system.

Exercise proved to be a frustration for Susan. Usually 20-30 minutes of aerobic exercise boosts mood. Susan's body could not tolerate strenuous exercise. She worked with a physical therapist to devise an exercise protocol, including yoga, and stretches for 5 - 10 min. a day. Too much exertion caused stress to the body that resulted in a day of bed rest, and at one point she was hospitalized after an intensive attempt at building up treadmill walking tolerance at her local health club. The therapist working alongside a CFS client must recognize the unique capabilities of each person to trust the body's wisdom.

Each individual needs to seek ways to make their dwelling a sacred space. Susan discovered that her mood lifted when she lit lavender candles, when she used a full spectrum light, surrounded herself with blankets, with cups of tea, and with peaceful music. She paid attention to the colors she wore, choosing to stay away from dark colors. She watched "happy" movies and TV. I recommended that she only briefly glance at newspapers and encouraged inspirational or frivolous reading. Susan sometimes could only read for short periods, due to difficulties in concentration. She tried to read each day. She brought me titles of books to read, from CFS sources to angel

and fairy books. Susan also cared for plants and the occasional neighbor-
hood cat. She began sewing small projects for the family members with a
great sense of accomplishment. This eventually expanded to creating purses,
wine bottle bags, and poodle skirts. She tried to maintain this healthy home
environment.

Depression can be isolating and it was vital for Susan to maintain
positive relationships. Fortunately, she had the support of her husband,
mother, sons, daughter-in-laws, siblings, grandchildren, friends, doctors,
and co-workers. Susan carried guilt about what she could not give in relationships. It was important for us to focus on what she COULD do and
speak from a position of gratitude. Susan began to acknowledge that her
illness provided opportunities for others to reach out and provide a loving
response. One of the favorite visualizations we used was the imagery of
being surrounded, like a blanket, by those who have been supportive, from
the former neighbor, to the first grade teacher, to store clerks, to waitresses,
to family members. Susan used this imagery to help on the "blue" days. The
memories help thwart isolation.

Susan had difficulty asking for help and being honest about how badly
she felt. She learned through the therapeutic process that it was ok to ask
for help when she needed it. I accepted her, whether or not she had makeup on, or if she had to be carried out of session, or not. She became more
accepting of the illness. Those around her, who loved her, became ok with
her having the illness. She could ask for help and it would be up to the
individual to decide. She need not make that decision. Family members
could learn to alter their expectations.

It was difficult for Susan to maintain relationships with colleagues
since her energy and mobility was limited. She tried to make periodic
phone calls or emails and was sometimes able to meet a colleague for a
meal. Susan and her husband gauged their social activities from "present"
planning, and limiting future engagements. This took much practice and
shifting. Susan is a methodical planner. She discussed these frustrations
and disappointments in session.

Susan experienced fear that she could not return to her career and her
former level of functioning. She remembered her high energy during the
long relapse period, but the difficulty with living in the present is that the

present pain and phase of the disease feels like it will last forever. We practiced relaxation exercises in sessions, including imagery to enhance "present" living. Meditation was rehearsed so that Susan could maximize focus and relax with her pain at home. Therapeutic art, and the use of pastels to promote non-perfection, enhanced the imagery sessions and provided an outlet for frustrations. The experience of creation can lighten the heart. I asked Susan to acknowledge three things daily for which she was grateful, and this helped bring life to a positive focus. Susan tried to resign herself to the notion that the future will happen, whether she worries or not, and she can choose not to worry. Each day can be a gift.

Another intervention used, at Susan's request, was editing. Because it was sometimes difficult for Susan to express complete thoughts and organize her writing, due to mental fog, she wanted me to review a letter to her physician. She was open to suggestions and was able to ask for the assistance. I encouraged her assertiveness and the articulation of her feelings.

This book is the ultimate example of therapeutic writing. Journaling, non-dominate hand writing, storytelling, and poetry were used to encourage self-expression. The use of the computer was sometimes easier than the physical exertion from writing by hand.

The involvement of Susan's husband was important to the process. Dealing with Susan's multiple hospitalizations and the care involved, produced family changes that needed to be processed. His added responsibilities in meal preparation, shopping, etc. caused manageable stress due to the strength of their relationship and their discussions about the effects of the illness. He chose to be proactive in her care, including seeking the latest research advances. He and Susan would share this information with me and with her team of physicians.

Susan reported that during her first bout with the illness, her children were teens and this proved challenging. They supported her by helping with daily chores and becoming more self-reliant. One son was in high school and the other son was just beginning his college life.

On a practical level, Susan requested, with the proper releases, that I fill out paperwork for her disability benefits. Prior to sending it out, I read it to Susan, making sure that I was not disclosing any information that *was uncomfortable. I also contacted physicians, with written releases, for continuity of care.*

I would like to offer a final note on the organization of my usual therapeutic session. I begin by lighting a candle, (with permission) which helps separate the therapeutic time from any other time in the day, and by offering decaf, water or tea. There are a soft blanket and pillows on the loveseat and I encourage clients to use them, if they choose. I want to project a feeling of nurturance. In the first session, confidentiality, office policies, background information and a psychosocial assessment are the focus. Preliminary goals are set. In the following sessions, we begin by addressing current concerns. Therapeutic interventions are gauged according to client needs. For example, I could tell by Susan's gait on the way to the office and by the tenure in her voice, how the session needed to proceed, given her energy level. It was vital for me to check my perceptions with her. We proceeded from Susan's cues. Sometimes home assignments were given, such as meditating five minutes a day. In closing the session, I ask the client to think of something positive, such as a wish, or a prayer, and blow out the candle. This closing ritual provides an uplifting end to our time together and an opportunity for another creation.

[Dr. Cherla and I mutually decided when it was a good time for termination of our Therapy Sessions. Therapy does not go on forever, but I do feel it is important to be able to schedule what I refer to as "a tuneup" whenever a patient feels it is needed.]

CHAPTER 19

GO TEAM GO!

Upon changing and adding new providers, my Medical Team has been working exactly as designed for the past fifteen years, and I feel I am receiving the best medical care available. Will I make changes in the future? Only if something begins 'not working', or if I find a new resource that could add to my treatment in a positive way.

You will discover later in this book, a chapter I added to determine when you might need to *assess your current medical team*, mapping the pros and cons for change. Then you will find a chapter with an *Eight Step Guide* for changing physicians. I have made changes in my string of pearls for differing reasons over the years, but never without weighing the positive and negative impact on my health.

Please understand that your medical team model may look different than the one I assembled. You should design a medical model to fit your own needs, that is, your own string of pearls!

It is understandable for the medical community to be frustrated and annoyed with the complexity of the Myalgic Encephalomyelitis (ME)/ Chronic Fatigue Syndrome (CFS) diagnosis, and the effectual inconsistency of symptomatological treatments. But it is not acceptable for the medical community to be frustrated and annoyed with ME/CFS patients.

Today I am extremely fortunate to have a great medical team surrounding me. However, it is important for you to know this did not happen for me until my second episode of ME/CFS. Unfortunately, many times it is when you are the most ill and incapable, that you need the most medical support. If you are too fatigued to pull together a group of medical professionals to meet your needs, enlist the help of a family member or a trusted friend to assist in your search.

As a patient you have the right to effective, ethical treatment. You have the right to be treated with respect and dignity. But, along with those rights comes patient responsibility. One of the most important responsibilities is providing your physician and entire medical team with detailed, consistent symptom information.

While this illness has no cure yet, best practice protocol remains in the hands of the medical community treating self-reported symptoms. It becomes very clear that **the recording of your symptoms with maximum detail and specificity, most certainly will improve the likelihood that you will receive the best tailored treatment for your unique set of symptoms.** This is in your complete control, and one of the most important things that you can do to assist in your recovery.

I have included in the following chapter a sample of the symptom charting that I have developed and have used with my medical team. It has evolved through two episodes of ME/CFS over a period of 30+ years. While you may feel free to use my format, please also feel free to adapt it to fit your own needs and symptoms.

I cannot emphasize enough the importance of personalizing your charts to meet *your* needs, identifying your specific symptoms, and continuing to revise your format to maximize it's use. It is important to remember, one of the confusing things about this illness; *We don't look sick!* For many persons around us, the graphic evidence on the chart is the only way they can see and get a feel for this disease.

CHAPTER 20

CHARTING OF SYMPTOMS AND PHYSICAL ENDURANCE

You will find the self-charting information can be used with multiple systems in addition to your medical team, during your quest toward reinstatement of health. It can be invaluable for use with your employer (be discreet with what and with whom you choose to share), for use with schools if the patient is a minor, unexpected emergency room visits, financial aid assistance (advisor/consultants, human service workers, etc.), with family members, and for disability reports and hearings.

Consider using the worksheet listing possible symptoms in Chapter 10 to identify the symptoms you want to chart. I advise using your worksheet to identify each and every symptom to share with your medical team, but then be selective in choosing the most severe symptoms for your daily charting. By "most severe symptoms" I mean those symptoms that are interfering with living your normal life. Which symptoms are keeping you from working/attending school, from regular exercise, from normal household functions, from family activities? The most severe symptoms will float to the top. You will recognize and become more clear about targeting those symptoms that are the highest priorities for your life.

Once you have completed your worksheet by yourself, or in consultation with your medical team, you are ready to design your own self-reporting charts. (See Self-Charting Examples near the end of this chapter.) You may find you have days when charting may be impossible due to the severity of your symptoms. I have learned to keep a month-at-a-glance calendar at my bedside to code chart using my own self-developed shorthand, until I could transpose it onto my official chart.

Another idea to consider is enlisting the assistance of a trusted family member or friend to maintain accurate charting for you when you are too weak, or when experiencing impaired cognitive functioning, or as I like to call it, 'brain fog'.

Through trial and error, I have learned that simplicity in design of your charting, and clarity in measurement, will increase the likelihood that even the busiest person on your medical team will value and actually use your charting as part of your medical treatment plan. It can be used to help direct medication trials, and as a guide for discontinuing protocols that are shown to be ineffective for your particular symptoms.

Tracking your progress during a medication trial is a most efficacious way of providing feedback to your Medical Team. I designed a more detailed Medication Trial Sheet that allowed charting of multiple doses per day. I then transferred the more detailed information to my regular monthly Self-Report Chart. The chart reflects my high/low energy levels for each day, with a 'on'/'off' code on the days I received the Ritilan dosage (see December 2003 Daily Chart near the end of this chapter). This can provide a Month-at-a-Glance self-report of the medication trial, and the patient's view of it's effect on their daily activities.

Charting will assist you in recognizing slow progress and honest personal effort that may otherwise be overlooked, clustering of symptoms, recognizing patterns of improvement/regression in different climate conditions, etc. I have been able to ascertain along with my medical team that I do not do as well in the hot, humid days of the mid-summer heat. I have been able to identify my months of progression lasting for longer periods of time, and my degrees of regression at a lower intensity the further into each episode. My medical team has consulted my charting for possible changes in medication dosage, tailoring best practice protocol, and suggested life style changes.

One month of self-report charting can provide your Medical Team a snapshot of your current condition. Multiple months of self-reports can provide valuable insight into the progression/regression of the illness, plus also provide details for medication trials. My main symptom was, and remains, fatigue, and my main goal was assessing and charting the timing of my own Post Exertion Malaise. Post Exertion Malaise (PEM) is the worsening of symptoms following even minor physical or emotional exertion, with symptoms typically worsening 12 to 48 hours after activity and lasting for days or even weeks. Thus, you will notice the main focus in my charting are my energy levels, with particular attention paid to energy levels following exertion of any type.

Fatigue was the main condition that prevented me from returning to work. It is so very important that you correctly identify your most severe and most debilitating symptoms to chart. Charting those symptoms that prevent you from achieving your normal day to day routine, can assist your Medical Team in providing the maximum relief from this chronic illness.

My charting evolved into to the following Progress Sheet Chart that I used with all of my doctors. I plotted it on graph paper turned sideways so I could capture an entire month on one sheet. This was not the first progress chart that I developed, but instead my final development was much refined. This led into looking at specific behaviors; behaviors that would lead to what I considered a return to normalcy for my life. It seemed to be more useful for my physicians, and was a quick snapshot of an entire month. My specialist always photocopied it and placed it in my medical chart in his office.

These charts include name, date of month and year, and patient number as an identifier number used by most doctor's offices and hospitals. The charts I am sharing range from the first week of my second episode May 21, 2001 through Feb. 2006. They reflect a month-at-a-glance of my life living with Myalgic Encephalomyelitis (ME)/Chronic Fatigue Syndrome (CFS). These are a few samples of those years: documentation of the gyrations of ME/CFS splattered across the graph paper that I had previously purchased for a happier use.

I developed this chart at the end of the very first week of my second episode. I was so scared and angry that my illness had returned. After all I had progressed from part-time return to work in Sept. 1990 until my current full time employment in May 2001.

I had worked eleven years! I quickly decided to start charting so I could recover and get back to work asap!

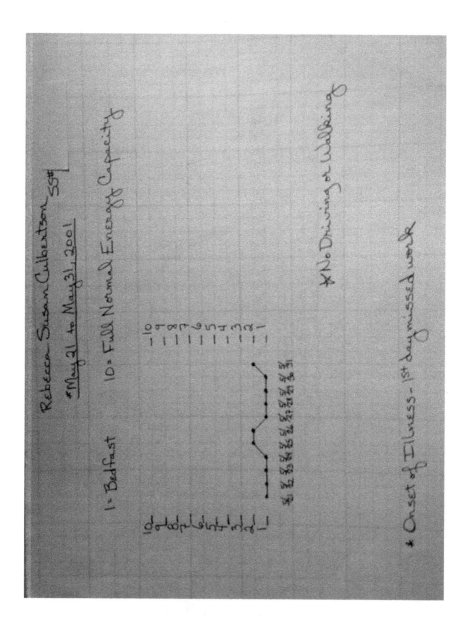

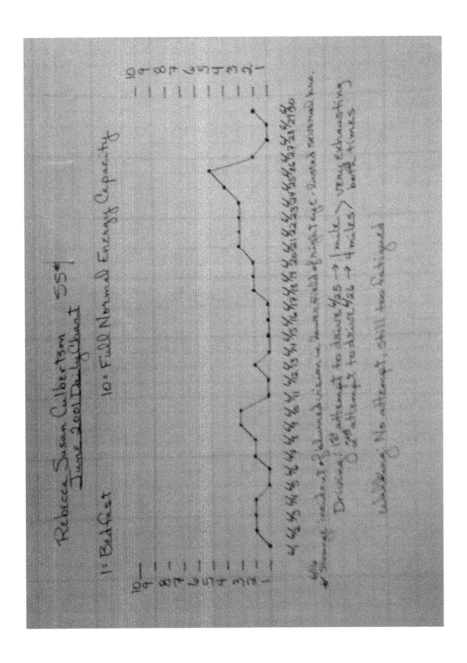

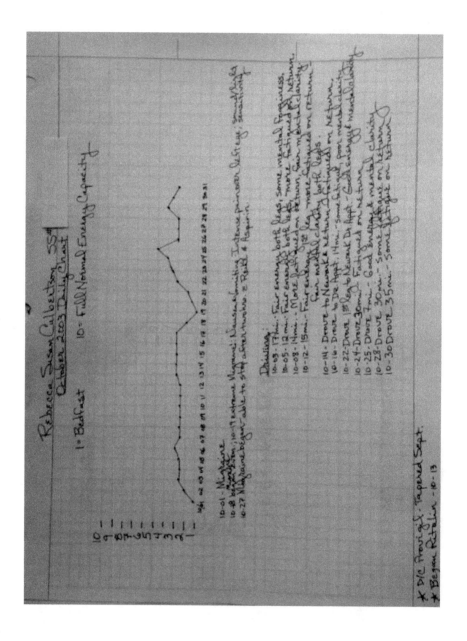

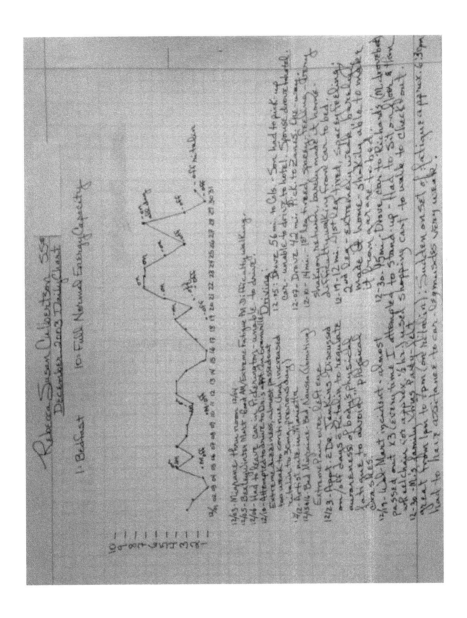

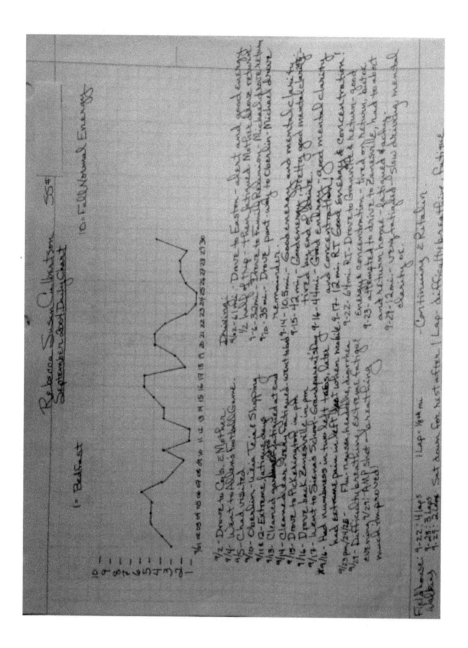

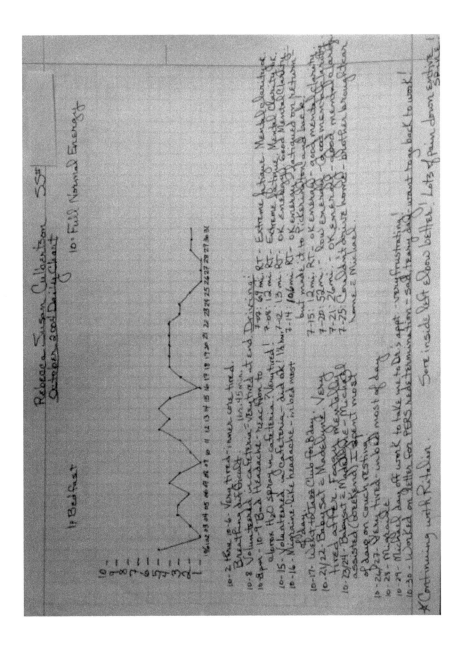

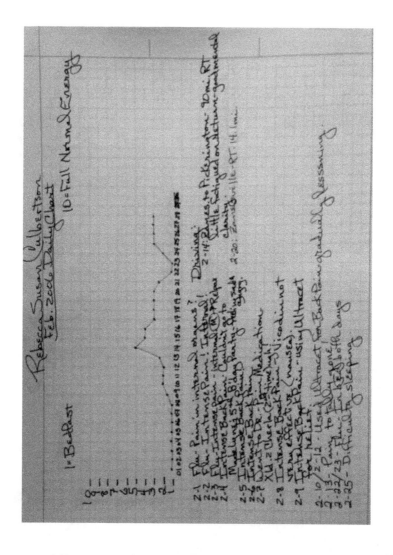

Just a follow up note to my charting, calling particular attention to October 2004 Chart, under "Driving:", with my charting dated incorrectly, prefixed with the July numeral "7", 7-07, 7-08, 7-12, etc.; instead of the correct October numeral 10-07, 10-08, 10-12. This was an extremely valuable, albeit unintentional charting displaying a mental mistake. Charting can reveal symptoms, duration of symptoms, efficacy of new treatments, etc., on a one page chart that can be handed to your physician; especially on days your mental and verbal skills are depleted.

CHAPTER 21

ASSESSING YOUR DOCTOR/PATIENT COMPATIBILITY

Hopefully you have found a good, solid doctor who is competent in treating Myalgic Encephalomyelitis (ME)/Chronic Fatigue Syndrome (CFS), or one who is curious and willing to try new ideas and treatments as they are discovered by the latest research programs. There is *nothing* more important to your health restoration than a good working relationship with your healthcare providers.

I think it bears repeating: It is understandable for the medical community to be frustrated and annoyed with the complexity of the ME/CFS diagnosis, and the inconsistency of treatments. But it is not acceptable for the medical community to be frustrated and annoyed with ME/CFS patients. No one *wants* to have this illness, and no one wants to cause frustration or annoyance for the medical community. Patients just want to regain their health and return to their former state of life.

I would like us all (patients and medical professionals alike) to consider a new, and I think most useful acronym that fits many chronic conditions generally, but fits ME/CFS particularly well:

MPF - Medical Provider Fatigue. While ME/CFS Medical Provider Fatigue (MPF) may not be an official condition, it has most certainly been a real situation in my personal experience - and the experience of other ME/CFS patients I have known. You can recognize MPF in your caregivers with subtle, and not so subtle expressions of frustration when treatment attempts fail to produce hoped for results. It is no surprise that caregivers can become discouraged with the long term and chronic recurring nature of ME/CFS. It is certainly exhausting to make repeated, well intended attempts that do not end in desired results. Even professional caregivers are at times victims of the, "Well, you don't look sick!" syndrome that friends and family too often exhibit. If you are constantly picking up on the non-verbal signals that you are just too much trouble, or not working hard enough for recovery, or worst of all, just pretending to be too tired to live your life, you are most likely dealing with a caregiver infected with MPF.

Some advice from personal experience: Give thanks you've spotted *their* problem, and politely move on. Medical Provider Fatigue in a caregiver has no known treatment or cure. *They've* got it and you don't have time or energy for it. So, just move on.

Over the years I have learned to identify medical community frustration, and you are probably already aware of the same or similar signs. You may also currently be suppressing your response to a medical provider as I have done in the past. I no longer ignore the signs of medical provider fatigue, as it is a valid detriment to the healing process. Plus, it can be a real contributor to patient hopelessness for recovery. And, it can lead to a reactive agitated depression.

EIGHT IDENTIFIERS OF MEDICAL PROVIDER FATIGUE (MPF)

Signs that I have witnessed myself include, but are not limited to, the following situations.

1. Looking down or writing/reading chart notes while you are attempting to give new ME/CFS symptom information.
2. Giving no response, or changing the subject immediately after you have given important information; in effect, dismissing in kind all contributions from you, the patient.
3. Total response limited to 'Uh-huh, Uh-huh, Uh-huh', with no follow-up questions or statements.
4. Lack of curiosity about new treatment literature and/or exploring new research.
5. Lack of interest in any new treatment or research ideas you present, no matter how legitimate the source.

6. Lack of ideas about potential next step treatment possibilities.
7. You feel you can not be really truthful with him/her (lack of trust).
8. Or, most egregious, glazing over in the eyes, even when you are giving brief, concise new symptom information.

STEPS TO PREVENT A DIVORCE FROM YOUR DOCTOR

Changing doctors can be very difficult. Extra stress with ME/CFS can cause symptoms to worsen, so I advise taking your time to consider this very important decision. You may want to discuss the situation with a trusted friend or family member to gain the advantage of another perspective.

Before changing physicians, or making any important life change I recommend mapping out a Pro and Con list as presented earlier in this book. I will share a sample list from my files, but please design your own to fit your particular situation.

PROS FOR KEEPING MY DOCTOR

1. Has history of my medical condition over the past 15 years.

2. Good if I have a flu or sore throat.

3. The office staff is very efficient and pleasant.

4. They have a good reputation in the community.

5. Doctor is pleasant after I mention ME symptoms.

6. The office is close to where I live.

7. _____

8. _____

9. _____

10. _____

CONS FOR KEEPING MY DOCTOR

1. Doesn't appear to listen to me.

2. Has refused (or ignored) new treatment ideas I have presented during a regular office visit.

3. I feel silly continuing to complain about the same symptoms, with no response from the doctor.

4. I am tired of being told that I just need to exercise.

5. Doctor is pleasant until I mention ME symptoms.

6. I would have to travel two hours round trip.

7. _____

8. _____

9. _____

10. _____

Remember, the previous chart is a chart I wrote for my own personal situation. You may not have *any* of the same issues in your situation. Write *your* pros and cons as they present with your own personal doctor.

Use all of the tools available to make a clear, concise decision. The weight of your answers in the Pro's and Con's List should not be weighted by the number of answers listed, but by the importance of the answer. It should be weighted toward the effect on your overall health.

If you decide to stay with your current doctor for now, you can always revisit this information, and go through the decision making process again later. However, do not place yourself in the position of staying with a non supportive, uninterested medical provider just because of your own anxiety about dealing with the situation. You could be harming yourself and your chances of recovery by remaining in a nonproductive relationship.

Finally, if you've established the pros and cons, and the pros outweigh the cons - BUT - it just doesn't **feel** right, go with your gut. A persistent bad feeling about your care provider no matter how good they look on paper should be heeded. If you consistently **feel** something is lacking, there is: your trust in your caregiver. In the end, the pro/con exercise is most useful when it sheds light on "why" you've been feeling the way you feel. The caregivers that are the most useful to you, bring you a sense of soothing and relief - even when they don't possess your favorite disposition or personality.

CHAPTER 22

EIGHT STEP GUIDE FOR CHANGING DOCTORS

If you have done a thorough assessment of your situation and you have made the decision to change physicians, it is important to next conduct the necessary research to find a new doctor. I have constructed an eight step guide that I use as a framework to assist me in making wise choices for selecting new caregivers. It is a good tool to assist with the avoidance of service duplication, finding a cohesive medical team, and finding the best fit for your particular healthcare needs.

During my first episode of Myalgic Encephalomyelitis (ME)/Chronic Fatigue Syndrome (CFS), I changed my doctor only one time. I was so overwhelmed with what was happening to me in the beginning, and then even more overwhelmed after my hospitalizations and surgeries, the thought of changing doctors never entered my mind. In fact, I remember a time of avoidance, of not wanting to *even think* about doctors. And then I heard Dr. Stephan Hanna from St. Joseph's Hospital on the radio in our living room. After being referred, diagnosed, and treated by his partner, Dr. Timothy Benadum, we happily drove four hours roundtrip for months to my St. Joseph's Hospital appointments with Dr. Benadum. I had found a physician that knew about my illness, believed in the diagnosis of Epstein Barre Virus (EBV, pre-ME/CFS term), and was providing his patients with the latest treatment regime known at the time. Perhaps equally important, he and the office staff believed me. They never gave me the sense that they doubted my self reported symptoms or that they suspected I might be malingering. I finally felt listened to, and heard.

After returning to full time work in 1990, I began to see a local physician for convenience reasons. I believed my illness was under control, and that I had defeated EBV, then known as Chronic Fatigue Syndrome (another pre-ME term). Not that my CFS was totally gone, but instead I had it under control, and I firmly intended to keep it that way. I had no knowledge that second or third episodes could occur, so I was operating under the impression that I would just continue to improve, and one day, like the flu, it would totally remit. There was virtually no information about this illness in the late 1980's, so I was flying blind with very limited research. Google and Siri were waiting in the wings to become a part of our everyday lives. Google became operational in Sept. 1998, and Siri had it's initial release on Oct. 4th, 2011. It seems now as though we have always had these resources - not so! Information is much more prolific and accessible today than just a few decades ago. We can take comfort and hope in that.

I changed primary care physicians (PCP) two times during my second episode for two entirely different reasons. My first change from the local physician that I hired after Dr. Benadum, was due to ME/CFS Medical Provider Fatigue, and their reluctance to work with my ME/CFS Specialist during my second episode. My PCP was showing signs of impatience with my forward, then backward progression in improvement. She became inattentive in diagnosing my non-CFS problems. She began questioning the process of forwarding my laboratory results to Dr. Hackshaw, as well as, negative comments about my ME/CFS specialist. After they proclaimed their opinion that my ME/CFS Specialist was in the medical business solely as a duplicator of services, for his own financial gain, I immediately decided to find another PCP.

But, I did so in an organized fashion. I began searching for a new PCP by researching the internet for doctors' ratings and reviews, by talking with family and friends about satisfaction with their providers, and I spoke with local hospital medical groups for a referral list of doctors in my area that were currently treating Chronic Fatigue Syndrome (CFS). After only two interviews I happily found a wonderful PCP as previously introduced in this book. My change to Dr.

Maria Jamiolkowski made a world of difference in my physician visits and in the coordination workings of my Medical Team Model!

The second change after ten years with Dr. Jamiolkowski was due to Medicaid/Medicare billing issues on the business side of her office. She prescribed a new medication for my deteriorating bone health, but as a stand alone provider she had limited services in billing options to assist me in payment subsidies. This created a major financial situation for me resulting potentially in thousands of dollars in out-of-pocket pharmaceutical costs. As an unfortunate consequence, I had to leave her care. She apologized for the limits of billing in her office, and encouraged me to find another point of care that could help me with my very real financial concerns. We parted amicably, and I changed to my current PCP, Dr. Ismet Ozkazanc, with noticeably little to no disruption in my PCP treatment.

The passing of medical records was smoothly accomplished as all charts were now in digital form and intra-connected through the local hospital system. My new PCP and my continuing Myalgic Encephalomyelitis (ME)/Chronic Fatigue Syndrome (CFS) Specialist, in a city over 50 miles away, were also interconnected by digital records, making the sharing of laboratory results and progress notes on both sides, accessible to the other. No more requesting, faxing, and signing releases of information on both sides, produced a seamless sharing of information. We were making progress! Welcome to the 21st Century. Now, if we could just find a treatment and cure for ME/CFS!

The following is an eight step guide I developed for myself, in an attempt to remain organized and calm during a stressful, but necessary process of changing doctors. Feel free to rearrange the steps, delete steps that do not relate to your situation, or add steps that you know would be conducive to your own personal process.

EIGHT STEP GUIDE FOR CHANGING DOCTORS:

STEP ONE: Talk with family and friends about the satisfaction with their current physicians. Word of mouth is one of the best methods for finding a competent, caring doctor. Equally important, if not more so, is to search out opinions from other ME/CFS patients and persons with other chronic, debilitating illnesses.

STEP TWO: Use online resources. There are many web sites that rate doctors by many differing variables, i.e., patient reviews, healthcare review standards, credentials, specialty areas, etc. Take your time and check out as many as possible - remember, this is not a race! This can increase the odds of finding the correct match for your medical needs.

STEP THREE: Hopefully, by this time one, two or three names will begin to top multiple lists. You may begin to hear the same name repeated multiple times. The old adage, "cream rises to the top" remains true. If this is not happening for you yet, repeat Step One using other medical sources, and repeat Step Two by expanding your data base to ME/CFS Support Groups, online ME/CFS blogs, etc. Laura Hillenbrand, the author of *Sea Biscuit* and *Unbroken*, has been a CFS sufferer since 1987, the identical year I became ill. She has varied information on her site from many contributors across the U.S. http://scopeblog.stanford.edu/2016/08/17/laura-hillenbrand-leaving-frailty-behind/. Much of this site is written by other ME/CFS sufferers in an informal 'comment' format. Her story is at: http://www.kenwilber.com/Writings/PDF/A_Sudden_Illness.pdf. It's worth checking out! Continue to explore until you have gathered enough information to feel comfortable in making a decision.

STEP FOUR: After you have made a choice of doctors, try ranking them in order of desirability. The very first thing to check after selecting your most desired provider is; do they accept your insurance carrier. You do not want to supplant medical stress with financial stress. If they do not, go to the second choice provider on your list, or explore the possibility of changing your insurance provider . [Do not change insurance until after the initial appointment.] You may discover while meeting face-to-face that this is not the provider for you, regardless of their illustrious credentials and/or glowing recommendations. It would be better to pay the initial appointment fee out of your own pocket than to change insurance providers and then, discover this is not the one for you!

STEP FIVE: Make an appointment with your newly selected provider. Make the appointment far enough in the future that gives you time to terminate from your current doctor, this also gives you time to collect your records from that office.

Be aware that some doctors may not be taking new patients. If you feel strongly about one doctor in particular, be willing to try to find a way to get referred. Some doctors will accept new patients only if they are a family member or friend of one of their current patients. Or they may be willing to place you on a waiting list. If you are placed on a waiting list, call the office weekly to check on your status. Do not call any more frequently - you do not want to become a pest to the office staff, as that could hurt your chances of being accepted as a new patient.

STEP SIX: After you have secured an initial appointment with your choice of a new doctor or group practice, immediately schedule an appointment with your current doctor. You need to be the one to alert your current doctor that you are moving to another physician for your future care. [If you already have a regularly scheduled appointment and plan to terminate at that time, just make sure your new doctor's appointment is sometime after that appointment date for chart transfer purposes. The smooth transfer of case records is an important concern and one you want to ensure during any transition.]

Depending on your new physician's office policy, they may prefer to have you sign their Release of Information Form and have your records transferred directly to their office. This is becoming the preferred method for transfer of records, as more and more offices have digital record systems.

STEP SEVEN: At your exit interview with your current doctor you should inform your doctor why you are leaving their practice. This will give them a chance to respond. They may be relieved that you are leaving, or they may request an opportunity to improve their service. The decision to stay or go will be entirely up to you - just be prepared if this situation occurs.

My advice is to write down your thoughts and reasons for making the change in your medical care. Write your doctor a letter. Reading it aloud at your appointment will give you the advantage of not having to remember the important points you want your doctor to know. [Remember, stress can cause mental confusion in ME/CFS patients.]

It is also fine to take a family member or friend with you for support. Make certain your support person clearly understands your reason for the exit visit, and the content of your letter. You do not want an unexpected reaction from your support person while terminating with your doctor.

If you feel too physically weak, or do not have the family/friend support you need, it is perfectly acceptable to terminate your doctor/ patient relationship via written document, posted to your physician. Remember to request the transfer of your chart to your new physician. You may have to make an in person visit to the business office to sign a release of information form. Be courteous and supply them with the new address, telephone and FAX numbers.

STEP EIGHT: The initial appointment with the doctor at the top of your list, should be treated like a job interview. Remember, you are the one doing the hiring! You are potentially hiring this person to take care of your health. If it doesn't feel right at the initial appointment, don't hire them. Go to the second, and third person on your list if necessary. Keep going until it feels right!

You are paying them to deal with a very frustrating and confusing illness. **Be up front about your own expectations and concerns.** Remember, as with your exit interview, write down your questions, or write a letter to your new physician and read it to them. ME/CFS causes mental confusion on the best of days. Stress will increase your mental confusion. Write it down!

Some basic questions that I have used in finding compatible physicians for my medical team are listed below. Please feel free to use any questions that may be relevant in your quest to hire a new physician. Include questions of your own that complement your personal situation and expectations. Remember to keep your list of interview questions as short as possible, without compromising your ability to make an informed decision.

Allow the doctor time to give thoughtful answers. Sort your most important questions to the top of the list, with the realization your session could be cut short by the physician being called to an emergency. And remember, you have every right to expect any physician to give your concerns their genuine consideration. Be picky, you are making a serious decision.

SAMPLE INTERVIEW QUESTIONS FOR HIRING PRIMARY CARE PHYSICIAN[*4]

1. Approximately how many patients have you treated with ME/CFS?
2. What do you know about ME/CFS, and do you believe ME/CFS is a real and valid illness?
3. Do you have a protocol for treating ME/CFS?
4. Would you be willing to work with my Medical Care Team?

Consider giving a copy of your Medical Care Team Model to the doctor with an explanation of each professional's role. You may use my sample model in Chapter 17 as a tool to develop your own model.

---

4 *Primary Care Physician (PCP) is a doctor for treating your medical healthcare. I use my PCP as a coordinating physician with my ME/CFS specialist, but you may use your PCP for both medical care and ME/CFS care if they are qualified and willing. In my own experience I have found it better to separate the PCP care from the ME/CFS Specialist care for reasons of medical fatigue and lack of ME/CFS knowledge.*

Consider giving the doctor a written copy of your expectations:

(a) You would be expected to share a copy of all my routine laboratory results with my ME/CFS specialist to eliminate duplication of service.

(b) You would receive a follow-up medical report after each visit from my ME/CFS Specialist.

(c) You could receive information from my psychotherapist if requested, with my written approval.

5. ADD YOUR OWN QUESTIONS AS DESIRED:

_____

_____

_____

_____

_____

Your goal should be to listen and to take notes. You can talk more at length about yourself at a later appointment. You really need to gather information so you can make an informed decision about whether or not to hire this person.

If the doctor indicates that they do not believe that there is such an illness, run, do not walk to the exit. Thank them for their time and leave. Go to the next doctor on your preferred physician list and repeat steps.

CHAPTER 23

SUICIDE SOUP

During my first episode of ME/CFS suicidal thoughts did not visit me. My younger son was in high school and still living at home. My parents were still active and supportive in my life. Plus, my illness began to abate after approximately three years. Looking back I believe our enhanced family structure, and the shorter length of illness were natural factors to the absence of this symptom.

During my second episode, I was alone at home most days during daytime hours while my husband was at work. My sons were married with children, and living their own busy lives, as they should. My father was now deceased, and my mother had been diagnosed with Alzheimer's. My illness had lasted, at this point in time, four years.

I experienced suicidal thoughts once during this second episode. I believe the more isolated environment, and the longer length of time of active debilitating ME/CFS symptoms had both contributed to the severity of my reactive depression and subsequent suicidal thoughts.

It was most interesting for myself as a therapist to experience what I consider to be the most alarming, dangerous state of mind a person can reach. Hopelessness.

This occurred with me about the 4th year mark. I believe this 4th year was poignant, as my first episode of ME/CFS lifted in the 3rd year of illness. I was subconsciously expecting the same timeframe for the resolution of this episode, and that wasn't happening. I was well into my 4th year of symptoms, and I wasn't experiencing the recovery that I had in my first episode of ME/CFS.

I actively worked with my therapist, Dr. Meisterman, on planning and preparing myself to deal with my increased depression during long winter months, etc. I actively worked with my disability mandated psychiatrist, Dr. Jenkins, on my distress over the length of time absent from my professional work environment. We worked on redefining my professional self; and the benefits of having ME/CFS. She actively assisted me with adjusting to the increased length of time this episode was lasting.

I questioned my ME/CFS Specialist, Dr. Hackshaw, why this episode was lasting so much longer than my first episode. He informed me that many times a second or third episode can last longer with more severe symptoms than a first episode. He also informed me I was older this time and that could be a factor. [At the onset of my first episode I was 39 years old, and at the onset of the second I was 53 years.] I replied, "Thank you so much for pointing that out". He smiled. I laughed.

Then I remember one afternoon in particular. I had been feeling sorry for myself. For some reason I didn't try to talk myself out of it as I usually did. This day I did not make myself think of all my riches - family, warm home, food to eat, etc., etc., etc. I jumped into my sadness with both feet. I didn't try to cheer myself. I was angry about my loss of health, loss of my professional self, loss of my ability to run every morning, loss of my dreams!

I began crying. I couldn't stop. Then I began sobbing. I couldn't stop. Then I heard a voice say, "Just kill yourself". Not my voice. Not my talking to myself voice. Not my voice. An unfamiliar voice that has not ever spoken to me again.

"The voice" startled me, scared me, and freaked me. I was so tired of fighting. I thought about the relief that death could bring.

Thankfully my thoughts and attention naturally diverted to the mental health training I had invested in so deeply. Even as I continued to sob, I began to review for myself, the information I knew to be true. As I had no plan for harming myself, and I just wanted these feelings of anguish to stop, I told myself "If you wait and breathe, these thoughts will go away". I repeated to myself, "This too shall pass."

I knew not to fight this crying, as tears actually release negative chemicals from your brain.[5] I knew to keep crying until it naturally stopped. Besides, I couldn't stop crying even if I tried. I knew I wouldn't cry forever, as it is physically impossible.

I turned on the television. It annoyed me. I turned it off. Upon discovering the TV was an irritant and had no effect on my continued sobbing, I stumbled to the kitchen and decided it was time to start dinner.....so, in my depressed stupor I did. Still sobbing, I entered the kitchen and retrieved veggies from the refrigerator. I put a large pot on the stove to catch my tear-stained ingredients. I remember chopping an onion and crying (this time not caused by the onion). {*I would not have picked up a knife if I had felt any inclination or had any thoughts of harming myself.*} Then I sobbed as I chopped carrots, celery and potatoes.

I ran research statistics about Golden Gate Bridge suicidal attempts over and over through my head as I cried.

According to 2005 estimated statistics, by 2012 there would be approximately a total of 1400+ suicide attempts from the Golden Gate Bridge since the recording began in 1937.[6]

As of the latest research stats only 26 persons have survived the jump. **All 26 survivors** when interviewed, reported the **same thought**

---

5 http://gibbsmagazine.com/CryinLaughing.htm
"Crying is a more complicated process than one at first would imagine. First of all, there are really three different types of tears. Basal tears keep our eyes lubricated constantly. Reflex tears are produced when our eyes get irritated, like with onions or when something gets into our eyes. The third kind of tear is produced when the body reacts emotionally to something. Each type of tear contains different kinds of chemical proteins and hormones. Scientists have discovered that the emotional tears contain higher levels of manganese and the hormone prolactin, and this contributes in a reduction of both of these in the body; thus helping to keep depression away. Many people have found that crying actually calms them after being upset, and this is in part due to the chemicals and hormones that are released in the tears."

6 http://en.wikipedia.org/wiki/Golden_Gate_Bridge#Suicides *According to 2005 estimated statistics, by 2012 there would be approximately a total of 1400+ suicide attempts from the Golden Gate Bridge since the recording began in 1937.*

as falling through the air, '**I wish I hadn't done this!**' [Summation of similar quotes.]

By the time my husband arrived home that evening, I had finally stopped crying.

I have never again had suicidal thoughts. If I had, I would have most certainly phoned my husband or Dr. Meisterman for help! I would not have ignored this symptom. Suicidal thoughts should never be considered unimportant. They need to be addressed at their first appearance.

If Suicidal thoughts remain, call 911 or your therapist immediately. Do not remain alone, call family or friends to stay with you until you are in the presence of a professional helper.

National Suicide Prevention Lifeline: 1-800-273-TALK(8255)

An absolute MUST for a person having suicidal thoughts: NEVER BE ALONE!

A suicide is rarely committed in front of others. It is usually a solitary act. If I had realized the thought that I was actively going to make an attempt, I would have dialed 911 for help. I would have phoned my husband, Dr. Meisterman or Dr. Jenkins on my Medical Team. There is a major difference between suicidal thoughts and an imminent suicidal attempt. However, I firmly believe that unresolved repetitive suicidal thoughts can most certainly lead to a suicidal attempt.

100% of suicidal thoughts are treatable, and can be resolved. I openly discussed my suicidal thoughts with my husband (who is also a therapist), Dr. Meisterman, and Dr. Jenkins. It is important, I firmly believe, to have at least one mental health specialist on your Medical Team during the active phase of ME/CFS.

I am including at the end of this chapter a list of Predisposing Factors to Greater Suicide Risk.[7]

By the way, the soup was ok, just a little salty.

_____

7   *https:sprc.org*
Major risk factors for suicide include:
Prior suicide attempt(s)
Mental disorders, particularly depression and other mood disorders
Access to lethal means
Knowing someone who died by suicide, particularly a family member
Social isolation
Chronic disease and disability
Lack of access to behavioral health care
Risk Factors Can Vary Across Groups
Risk factors can vary by age group, culture, sex, and other characteristics. For example:
Stress resulting from prejudice and discrimination (family rejection, bullying, violence) is a known risk factor for suicide attempts among lesbian, gay, bisexual, and transgender (LGBT) youth.
The historical trauma suffered by American Indians and Alaska Natives (resettlement, destruction of cultures and economies) contributes to the high suicide rate in this population.
For men in the middle years, stressors that challenge traditional male roles, such as unemployment and divorce, have been identified as important risk factors.
PTSD, post traumatic stress disorders (military & rape traumas, for example).

CHAPTER 24

A MAJOR BREAKTHROUGH: PROS & CONS OF MYALGIC ENCEPHALOMYELITIS / CHRONIC FATIGUE

The personal reckoning of having experienced an episode of suicidal thought was the push I needed to consider Dr. Jenkin's repeated attempts to get me to put into writing the Pros and Cons of my ME/CFS diagnosis. Prior to this episode, I couldn't, or wouldn't, allow myself to consider that there could ever be *anything* positive about having this disease. I since have come to appreciate this exercise, as this process began the reframing I needed to move forward with my life. I can now add the *pro* of having had the time to write this book that I would not have had, if I had been working at my mental health job!

The *cons* were easy for me - loss of income, loss of professional self, loss of health, etc. The *pros* took longer to uncover; but as I identified each one it became easier to deal with the losses. I now fully appreciate having had more time to spend with family. I remind myself I had unlimited time to spend with my Mother as she progressed through the stages of Alzheimer's. I can have lunch with one of my sons, Jon or Chad, or coffee and treats with my grandchildren, Allen, Kelsey, Siena, or Madelyne. I can have travel time with my retired spouse, Michael. I can babysit my great-grandchild, Archer, when I am able. None of this would be possible if not for the change in my lifestyle due to this illness.

Use the chart below to begin your own consideration, as you are ready. Hopefully it will not take you as long as it took me to identify the pros of having ME/CFS. With having this chart available, you will as least have the advantage of recognizing when a *pro* is realized and you can quickly document it on your chart until you have enough listed to make the switch in your mind. I encourage you to trust that this exercise, no matter how difficult at first, can and will prevent anger from building to a negative tipping point. This can also be used as a Family Exercise where everyone can chart from their viewpoints, and then be discussed among family members. This can assist in the helplessness that most family members feel in dealing with a loved one's illness.

I remain eternally grateful to Dr. Jenkins for not giving up on me, and continually encouraging me to find the positive side of my illness. Sorry for having taken so long, Dr. Jenkins!

PROS OF HAVING ME/CFS:	CONS OF HAVING ME/CFS
1. _____	1. _____
2. _____	2. _____
3. _____	3. _____
4. _____	4. _____
5. _____	5. _____
6. _____	6. _____
7. _____	7. _____
8. _____	8. _____
9. _____	9. _____
10. _____	10. _____

CHAPTER 25

DEALING WITH LOSS

It is difficult to know where to begin when dealing with the issue of loss in regards to Myalgic Encephalomyelitis (ME)/Chronic Fatigue Syndrome (CFS). The illness has so many tentacles that touch every single aspect of your life. We have already dealt with several areas in previous chapters, but it is difficult to think of any area of your life that this illness does not affect.

We have looked at multiple areas of loss in one's life attributed to ME/CFS; such as, loss of professional identity, loss of income, loss of ability to exercise, loss of driving, which can lead to loss of independence, loss of financial security, and, most importantly, loss of overall health and well being.

Losses that we haven't yet discussed are no less important. They may be more subtle, often unspoken losses, but often are just as devastating as those mentioned previously. The loss of self confidence, loss of friends, loss of ability to maintain intimacy, loss of ability to parent adequately, loss of ability to express one's creativity, and after multiple hospitalizations, testing and doctor's examinations, modesty can even be taken away.

How do we manage our mental healthiness when we expend so much energy just by bathing, getting dressed, brushing hair, arranging transportation to go out, walk to our destination (already feeling exhausted) and are told by the first person we bump into, "You don't look sick!" How do you hold onto your self confidence, and not just want to go home and climb back into bed? How do you control your anger and hurt feelings? How do you go on? There are no easy answers, but there are ways of managing your own internal thoughts that can help prevent any further decline of your self confidence.

It is vastly more important what you tell yourself, than what another person says to you. I will often translate, *"Well you don't look sick!"* into *"That person really doesn't understand ME/CFS, and how hurtful that comment is"*. Then I attempt to say "Thank you!", and move on quickly. I send a blessing out to the universe mentally saying, "May this person never know a chronic illness". Thoughts travel through your mind on the same neural pathways as the spoken word, so therefore you do have control over what you allow to enter your consciousness.

Although it is very important to stay positive and "future think", it is also important to be realistic with your internal thoughts. It is easy after say a stretch of nine or ten good days (especially if consecutive), to know that you are feeling stronger and you have the desire to make future plans, (i.e., tomorrow I will do laundry, let's meet on Tuesday for lunch, yard work on Friday). Then the ME/CFS reminds you of it's presence - crushing fatigue, mental disruption, pain in every joint, etc., etc., etc.

It is your job to learn to ride the roller coaster with as little emotional disruption as possible. The energy you do have is best used toward recovery, not wasted on frustration. It is a mindset change, not an easy thing to accomplish, but also not impossible!

The ups-and-downs and wild turns create not only a "roller coaster" for you, but also for your close family and friends. I am not suggesting an emotional shut-down; what I am suggesting is an opportunity to learn to redirect your energy only toward positive thoughts. Research has shown the best predictor of any type of success has a direct correlation to the degree of positive attitude exhibited by the person being tested.

As you begin this transformation from your usual negative thought, mine being "Oh no! Here it comes again!", to a new more positive thought, "I better rest now so I can get through this smoother and faster!". Again I remind you, I am not suggesting an emotional shut-down. I am, however, suggesting that you pass through the frustration and pain as quickly as possible.

I have included several options for Negative Release Exercises at the conclusion of this chapter. Over time I have been able to shorten my negative frustration time, and have found my return to positive energy smoother and more fluid with practice. I cannot proceed without including a precautionary note that we all advance in our own time. No two fingerprints are the same, and no two negative transformation times are the same.

We all have our own unique path and method to recovery. We must be kind to ourselves during the times of frustration and personal anguish - sometimes will be more difficult than others, and that's ok! The important thing is to just keep trying, and doing the best of which you are capable.

NEGATIVE RELEASE EXERCISES

1. Journaling - Writing down your thoughts, negative or positive, can be a valuable tool in your daily effort to release negative emotional content. It can be surprisingly useful to keep a daily "Appreciation Log" where you record at least three things, people, circumstances, abilities, etc. that you sincerely appreciate. Research has shown that we have the same thoughts day after day. In fact, as high as 98% of our thoughts may be repeated day after day. Change your thoughts, change your life!

2. Emotional Release - Do not ignore or stifle your body's natural response to stress. It is not a weakness, but a strength, to recognize when your body desires to release stress through tears, verbal expression, or even screaming. Preferably not screaming AT another person, but productive screaming as an outlet of emotion, directed mentally at your chronic illness in a private place where your inhibitions are not in check.

3. Music - Yes, music can soothe the soul. Passive listening can be achieved even on your most physically limiting days. Active participation, if you are so gifted or so bold, can be an ultimate spirit lifting experience even on your most "down" day. Select your genre carefully, find what is right for you, from rock to

classic, this is a very personally tailored emotional release that anyone can achieve in the privacy of your own home.

4. Candles - I find lighting one candle or more can help pull me out of a "dark" day. If you are bedfast, keep a candle on a bedside table within easy reach. I have found unscented candles are best for me, as scented ones can sometimes set off a migraine episode. However, if you have a favorite scent, indulge in the olfactory pleasure until your spirits are lifted! Battery powered candles are a nice worry free choice.

5. Tailor a Plan for yourself - list other negativity releasers that you find personally cleanse both your negativity and repetitive self defeating thoughts. While you may not be able to change your illness (at least this very instant), with determination and practice you can get pretty good at changing your mood. Aim for soothing, not final solutions. Often there is significant satisfaction in achieving some relief, even when you know you can't totally resolve an issue. Relief and soothing, "Ah, that's better".

CHAPTER 26

THE IMPORTANCE OF HAVING A PERSONAL SUPPORT SYSTEM

I truly cannot say enough about the difference family and/or friend support can make in dealing with Myalgic Encephalomyelitis/Chronic Fatigue Syndrome or any chronic illness. The ME/CFS diagnosis permeates every relationship the ME/CFS patient has. It may be difficult for family[8] or friends to remain empathetic and understanding month after month of this prolonged confusing illness. After all "we don't *look* sick".

It is imperative for your personal support system to receive information about ME/CFS, and to continue their education as new symptoms appear, as the illness ebbs and flows, and during long periods of stagnated progress.

Support in the early stages will probably feel no different than your support system would be for any other diagnosis. ME/CFS patients report waning support as the illness drags on. Divorce rates are reported to be as high as 75% when one partner has a chronic illness. Just when a person needs extra support and understanding is usually when the relationship falls apart.

The ending of a relationship whether by divorce or separation of partners, touches so many other parts of a person's life. Moving from a couple to single hood while dealing with ME/CFS, adds greatly not only to financial stress, but also a myriad of other personal complications.

---

8   *I use the term "family" to include "chosen family" even if not biological or by legal definition.*

I am so very fortunate to have had a partner and family members that were supportive with me from the very beginning of my illness. I do not know from actual life experience what it takes to deal with a spouse or parent with ME/CFS. I do know it has made a major difference in my life that my spouse, Michael, and my sons, Chad and Jon, did everything possible to make me feel loved and accepted during my long illness.

[My spouse, Michael McVicker, will be concluding this chapter to give voice to one family's struggle in finding a path through this frustrating illness of ME. He is the expert in coping with a family member diagnosed with a chronic illness, plus an expert with the added difficulty of a blended family raising teenagers. He acted and writes through the lens of a mental health professional with over 40 years of experience. He has my eternal gratitude and admiration for his unorthodox, humorous methods of familial support throughout my illness. Whatever it was, it worked! My sons love him, and I am so graced and nourished by his total support.

If only every family could understand this illness as families understand and support family members with cancer or heart disease, it would enhance an ME sufferer's life beyond our greatest hope."

Please note Michael uses the lower case i in his writings to distinguish his voice from mine in this continuing chapter. I highly recommend sharing his voice with your family.]

A VIEW FROM THE SIDELINE
by Michael McVicker, OCPSII

i have put off writing this for over a decade and a half. Susan first asked me to "write something" addressing the impact of ME/CFS on family members and caregivers nearly 17 years ago. My procrastination has risen to Olympic proportions in those passing years. It wasn't until doing a final edit of this book - which i highly recommend - that i slammed heart first into the primary reason for my profound resistance to "write something".

As i was making a focused conscious effort to read every word she had painstakingly put into this book, i came to her amazing handwritten charts in Chapter 20. While reading the history of her struggle with this wretched illness, i was doing pretty well recalling events and milestones of the journey with a sufficient degree of objectivity and operative emotional distance. (After all, i was doing a necessary chore of editing and attempting to keep my adoration of this heroic woman in reasonable proportion.) Until i slammed into those handwritten charts! Objectivity and emotional distance ended. Those dates, those graph lines, those notes, especially those very personal notes, crushed me.

A thick, heavy blanket of subjectivity dropped over me. i was back in it! No distance, no distraction, no possibility of denial or comforting distortion. Suddenly, i was smothered in fear, confusion, and fierce anger; surprisingly unprepared to be suddenly so sad.

My procrastination now made easy sense. i wanted to stay away from all of that emotional crap. i wanted to defend the refuge of my hard gotten defense mechanisms. They had taken years to develop. i was hiding. But enough about poor me.

I would like to say a few words about those brilliant handwritten charts. They are invaluable for the patient, for the doctors (and other professional caregivers), for employers, and for family and close friends. Invaluable for all who struggle to understand this strange, life altering illness. i frankly do not know how Susan thought to do this charting, nor how she physically, mentally or emotionally managed to make the daily entries. I'm a tiny bit proud to report that "i helped" from time to time. Keeping those records current has proven its value repeatedly. On the difficult days, pitching in to keep the record clear and current is a valuable contribution a caregiver or family member can offer.

My appreciation for the power and usefulness of these charts grew enormously, after witnessing the consistently positive response having graphic evidence received from physicians, nurses, therapists and even attorneys. Having evidence of duration and intensity of impairment, along with brief understandable descriptions of notable days made a significant difference in the professional's perception, and in the way Susan got treated.

i would also call the reader's attention to the chart dated October 2004. On this chart Susan has transcribed notes from a bedside journal to further detail and explain the raw data on the graph. Her notes had the appropriate daily dates, but had incorrectly recorded the month for those days. A clear example of mental fog. i reviewed the notes and they matched my recollections for that timeframe. October is her birthday month. Not being able to properly celebrate birthdays and other special events is just one of many memorable pains in the *arse* which ME/CFS imposes. That "brain fog" stuff is a real deal. Again, i don't think i can overstate how important this documentation can be. Like those overpriced shoe people say, "Just Do It!".

THE DEFINITIVE GUIDEBOOK TO BEING A GOOD PARTNER FOR THE SUFFERER OF ACUTE DEBILITATING ME/CFS

It's Pretty Simple:

- FIGHT through the overwhelming FEAR & CONFUSION
- WRESTLE your profound ANGER into some sort of moment to moment submission
- Find anyway you can to SOOTHE your SADNESS (At least enough to keep it from descending into an agitated clinical depression)
- Lastly, find and NUTURE YOUR SENSE OF HUMOR (You're going to need it)

Now you're pretty much set to........
MAKE IT UP AS YOU GO!

It really is fairly simple. Unfortunately,
Simple often ain't all that Easy.

For me, the truth is, there is no official guidebook. i am left to report my reflections of how we, as a couple and a family survived, and i believe, thrived through it all. Once we recognized whatever this was, was very very serious, and it was not going away on its own; i launched into six months, or more of frantic searching for definitive answers. i fairly quickly recognized that i would settle for reasonable explanations.

For me, those early months were a tight wire act of trying to manage the ebb and flow of my chronic state of panic. After we settled into some reasonable assurance that whatever this was, *(remember, doctors were as perplexed as we were),* was not going to kill Susan, just inflict interminable confusion and suffering, my panic settled. Now i could give fuller attention to my angry depression and a far more steady state of chronic anxiety. The mountain of unknowns was sometimes maddening. Susan and i were "solution seekers" by both trade and disposition.

After coming to a grudging recognition that a non-negotiable chronic illness had moved into our home, the next order of business was doing everything possible to keep ME/CFS from imposing itself too deeply upon Susan's two sons, my wonderful step-sons. What a glorious gift she had chosen to share with me. Doing right by them, scared the *"ship"* out of me. Still more pressure to cuddle close with anxiety, confusion, and increasing uncertainty - and we danced on - all four of us together.

At the onset of Susan's initial episode of ME/CFS, Jon, our oldest boy, was blossoming into a young adult and was a bona fide basketball star. He earned All-Ohio honors, and incidentally was recently inducted into his High School's Athletic Hall of Fame. Although i most admire his providing us with three lovely Grandchildren, and a Great-Grandson! By far, Jon's most impressive accomplishment is what a solid and loving parent he has become. Jon was living with his biological Father when his Mother became so suddenly ill. He was transitioning to his University living, and Susan made it very clear a major priority was doing everything possible to keep her mystery illness from becoming an emotional impediment to Jon's progression into early adulthood. My contribution was to support her choice to ensure he worried as little as possible about his Mom. i truly don't know how well we succeeded. i do know Jon managed to get on with his dive into adulthood, and he is now successful in love and life and parenthood (now also, grandparenthood); with all the unforeseen challenges that brings.

And then there's our younger boy, Chad, who was just starting high school when his Mom fell ill. We were fortunate, in some happy ways, Chad was a bit more mature than his years. Through his junior high school timeframe he had witnessed his Mother and i presenting several Training Seminars for a range of professionals. He had also helped in organizing handout materials, and was comfortable and capable in assisting with the mechanics of seminar etiquette. He had also proved himself to be an asset when we lived in the apartment above Susan's private therapy practice. A living arrangement that made it possible to afford the facility cost of the business that i had just joined. We were an odd sort of family/ step family business!

In short, any possible shields were down for Chad. Again, my major contribution, beyond emotional support and technical advocacy for his Mother, was to find a way to assist Chad through the minefields of this frightening, often dramatic chronic illness. So i did the only thing i could think of - i sort of forced the kid into being my playmate. At the time, this was not a conscious well thought out strategy. It's just the rhythm we slid into in order to survive the HEALTH BOMB that had exploded into our seriously happy collective life.

My earliest memory of Chad is still one of my most vivid. It involves a fully loaded chili, onion, cheese and relish foot long hot dog. Chad was nearly eleven years old and we had gone to a local "Dog & Burger" joint he liked, so his Mom could introduce him to this weird guy she was dating. (It was not lost on me that if i failed to receive the kid's stamp of approval, any prospects of continuing my relationship with his Mother would be seriously impaired; although Susan was kind enough not to say so out loud.)

Chad had yet to manifest the freakish adolescent growth spurt that was to catapult him to the disturbing height of 6'3". He and his older brother try to be taller than the other to this day. i can't see much actual difference in their "too tallness", but it's still fun to provoke them about this vital height issue. It is a true joy for me that the Brothers remain genuinely close and truly enjoy spending time together as their busy adult lives evolve. Meanwhile, back to that overloaded foot long.

This then smallish nearly eleven year old, sitting beside his Mother and directly across from me, lifted his foot long hot dog like a long rifle to his face, paused dramatically before his initial bite, fixed me with an unmistakable glare and said forcefully to me, " Stop leering at my Mother!". Thus our relationship was defined - it was on! (By the way, I've yet to stop leering at his Mother, and he's recalled his restriction.)

By the time of Susan's initial frightening and sudden episode of ME/CFS, Chad and i were getting along well. He was used to my being a regular component of his transportation to multiple school activities, and, of course, the local mall and movies, as well as, 4-H activities. 4-H was a vibrant part of his connection with his biological Father, and that larger extended family system. We had worked out early on that "i wasn't his Real Dad". Still, i was important enough to his transportation needs and his next pair of absolutely essential and extravagantly over valued "Jordan's" (at the time, the only acceptable footwear), that i remained relevant in his life. Besides, we both enjoyed playing together and i believe he caught on quite early that i was just stupid devoted to his Mom. We were doing alright working out the blended family stuff. When ME/CFS forced itself into our lives, we had already learned to play and laugh together. This would become a very welcome and unexpected source of relief and comfort - at least for me.

There were, of course, some very troubling times when we had no idea what was causing Susan's utter and terrifying collapse. At the dramatic onset of Susan's illness, i feel quite certain i completely failed to pay enough attention to either of our boys. i was giving every spare moment to controlling my own sense of raging panic.

This was particularly true during Susan's twelve nightmarish days of exploratory hospitalization and subsequent, needless surgeries. A furious and anxious timeframe when we learned so much about what this dreadful illness WAS NOT. Her "diagnosis of exclusion" was to be a grueling, and i still believe, nearly deadly process. Those were twelve terrifying days of hospitalization when she was flattened and deeply exhausted, and still being poked, prodded, stuck and bled, x-rayed, imaged in technically perverse ways and injected with toxic chemicals, awakened after any moment of sleep she could snatch.

She was so fatigued she was unable to eat (she lost 15 pounds in twelve days, and she barely topped 100 pounds when they began testing her) - i was a MESS. And by this time in my life, i was one of those guys that folks came to, hoping to find professional help with their own mess.

i remember what seemed like an endless parade of white coated specialists, each with their own white coated gaggle of aspiring physicians-to-be following behind. It seemed each time a specialist failed to identify "the problem" and passed her off to the next Specialty, Susan got weaker and thinner. A terribly high price to learn what wasn't wrong with her.

Looking back, i barely gave a thought to the medical bills that were mounting and well beyond our ability to pay. Dealing with that pesky detail would command our attention a little further on in our journey through the medical minefield. Again, i am fairly certain i was mostly useless to Jon and Chad during this taxing period.

i do clearly remember being unspeakably grateful to Susan's parents who did not hesitate to step in and keep Chad's routine as little disturbed as possible during that time. They also propped me up both mentally and emotionally more often than they could have possibly known. It is impossible to overstate the importance of their help.

Later, when the frenzy of finding out "What it Wasn't" had become more cognitively and emotionally manageable, i somehow got Susan's Private Practice customers contacted and linked to appropriate and reliable therapy options. With regret and remorse, i saw to the final details of closing down the cherished Family Practice Susan had worked so hard to establish; the Practice i was so very flattered and excited to have recently joined. i had left a long held outpatient therapist position at a local Mental Health Agency. i was now out of work, madly in love, responsible for a young adolescent and his Mother, who was now critically ill with a mysterious illness.

It is only with hindsight that I can see, and more vividly feel, a very peculiar sort of grief at the loss of Susan's rapidly growing Private

Practice. Establishing and marketing a successful psychotherapy practice is a significant accomplishment. The loss of that Practice, in which i had a committed investment, added a considerable weight of grief to the already formidable burden of this confusing illness. The massive turmoil ME/CFS was churning in our lives disguised a strange kind of grief that simply had to be set aside at that time.

With the loss of the Practice and the office CLOSED we were now faced with the pressing need to find alternative housing; preferably in our younger son's current school district. Happily we found an old farmhouse outside of town, in the district Chad preferred, and it was in our price range - cheap! Although i was soon to learn of the unfriendly cost of fuel oil in a rustic old farmhouse with little to no insulation. We were running on fumes; broke; with a heavy load of unexpected (unimaginable really) medical bills and living off the remains of meager savings and growing credit card debt. "Pressure Soup" with an uncomplimentary "Side Salad of Stress" was being served with every meal - whether you wanted it or not.

We had gotten moved into our "new to us" house and Chad's life was in a more or less steady rhythm. Susan's health was severely compromised and she was confined to bed the majority of days, or on the first floor couch if both Chad and i were absent. While she was still profoundly ill, often in pain and nearly always incomprehensibly weakened; we had seen incremental progress. She wasn't exactly getting a lot better but she seemed to have stopped getting worse. i still awakened once or twice a night and observed her closely to make sure she was breathing.

Disturbingly, we still had no idea of why she was ill or what could be causing this misery. However, we had begun to hear of other people, usually young hardworking professionals, mostly women - who were having similarly horrible experiences. i remember feeling a bit callous at the tiny speck of twisted hope that came with hearing we might not be the only family dealing with whatever this was. i'm pretty sure i never told Susan that. We were unbelievably starting to settle into this new state of chronic uncertainty. The only thing i was sure of, "it takes a whole lot of money just to stay broke". i really needed a job.

Most unexpectedly, i received an offer to become the Interim Clinical Director of a Residential Treatment Facility. A decision on the offer needed to be made quickly. The facility was located 40 miles from our new housing and would mean routine 10 hour days in addition to travel time - occasional evening and weekend hours were also likely.

The facility served troubled adolescents from a six county area and the place was undergoing turbulent organizational changes of its own. Ordinarily this would be an ideal opportunity to do the kind of work i actually loved. A challenging uncertain situation that would require energetic creativity. However, taking this vocationally and financially attractive position would mean far more time away from Susan and Chad than i was even nearly close to being comfortable with. Conflicted and scared, i accepted.

[Once again i want to be extremely clear; accepting that job would have been impossible without the loving support and capable help of Susan's parents and extended family, who fortunately lived close by.]

This job clearly saved us financially. Hindsight now allows me to recognize a then under appreciated advantage of that very challenging position. It provided powerful moment-to-moment distractions that, upon reflection, truly soothed my then obsessive anxiety about things at home. Clearly not a cure; and yet at that time the urgent but actionable vocational problems were a surprisingly welcome relief. The problems at work were of both an administrative and therapeutic nature. Almost always acute and urgent and requiring decisive response. More stress? More pressure? Yes.

The joyful difference between work stress and the stressors that cling to ME/CFS is simple: the new job came with fairly substantial responsibilities and expectations AND the authority and means to make critical decisions. A big bonus was that even less - than - optimal decisions could be reviewed and improved.

Work stress was blissfully acute, often recurring, and temporary.

At home we faced chronic fatigue, fatigue beyond tired, fatigue that slept with you all night but never rested and left you more exhausted upon awakening than the night before, fatigue that had moved in to stay, fatigue that really meant Chronic Relentless Uncertainty and Stress. A different creature altogether.

i believe it was during this tense period of life that i internalized (perhaps only unconsciously, instinctively then) how very important even a little relief and soothing can be in the face of chronic conditions beyond your control. Even intense acute stress is made doable by the knowledge that a solution exists and can eventually be found. i also want to call attention to the dynamic nature of "responsibility - expectation - and authority" when dealing with chronic external stresses.

Caregivers often accept very reasonable responsibility and expectation when they enter a caregiver relationship - both personally and professionally. It just goes with the territory. Where it gets tricky, sticky, and downright icky is when any caregiver imposes exaggerated INTERNAL EXPECTATIONS upon themselves. Self imposed expectations beget responsibilities beyond even the most loving and well meaning caregivers ability to deliver. The temptation to do this is many times irresistible. All sorts of "YUK!" come of this temptation. You can't help yourself from becoming a part of the problem. Most times it's so sincere and subtle you don't notice you've broken a Caregiver Boundary.

Professional Caregivers often surrender their "professional" status when they blindly slide across the boundary between paid employee and become an unwitting volunteer. It eventually will complicate and diminish care.

Loving and caring for a person with any chronic illness is a long term project. A journey with an uncertain destination. There are, oh, so many unforeseen twists and obstacles, even some tender and cherished surprises. So, i most sincerely encourage you to put your attention on "soothing" and "simple small reliefs" when hopeless feelings flirt with you.

i carry a fierce appreciation for that Adolescent Treatment Facility job to this day - for a great many reasons. The biggest drawback was being too far, too long, and too often away from Susan and our boys. Those drives to and from work were commonly so preoccupied with worry that i could not recall the actual drive. My unconscious mind proved to be a swell driver because my conscious thoughts were focused on the farmhouse, not the road.

i am resolutely certain that Susan's health and our situation in general would have been far far worse without the love, support and ongoing assistance of family. Susan's family never doubted the seriousness of the mysterious illness that had befallen her. They were well acquainted with her, "I'll do it myself, Thank You", workaholic, overachiever type personality. While i know they were often baffled and afraid, they never wavered in their commitment and eager willingness to help us. Her parent's emotional support, physical presence, and frequent crockpots of soup were essential to maintaining our quality of life during that critical timeframe of Susan's initial episode of ME/CFS. It truly is impossible to overstate the importance of having that unshakable Family Support Network!

If you should find yourself suddenly drowning in the tidal wave a major health crisis can bring, i urge you to both **ask for and accept** help at the earliest possibility. Asking for and gracefully receiving help seems so sensible and self evident as i write this. Only looking back into the jaws of that suffocating confusion, fear, and at times outright panic can i recognize the dumbfounded paralysis that can seize you. It did me - for a while. And that brings me back to Chad.

With Jon off exploring the wonders and challenges of higher education at "The" major university in our area, we were pleased he had taken a major step forward into adulthood. We (Susan, Chad and myself) then focused on settling into a very different life at our farmhouse. Being private and affordable, fuel oil cost aside, were major advantages. Being without air conditioning on a working sheep and pig farm, less advantageous. There were hot summer days when the olfactory intrusion was more problematic than the summer heat. But the landlords who operated the farm were dependable, kind and provided the comfort of being close by if Susan should ever need quick assistance. Thus, out of immediate financial jeopardy and Susan still bed fast most days, but making incremental improvement, we proceeded to nestle in as best we could. We continued to be supported by

Susan's core and extended family. Our little subunit was in the process of defining a peculiar new normal.

It took Susan several months before getting strong enough to clearly register and begin coping with the radical circumstances that had befallen us. i do realize i often speak of "us" and "we" many times while being very clear it was Susan that was being smashed and tortured by this Mystery Plague. You don't need a background in Family Therapy to recognize such a sudden major chronic illness makes a HUGE SPLASH in any family pond. The ripples are going to roll on to the extreme edges of the pond.

Professionally, i had witnessed even less intense and less dramatic events leave a mark on many extended family members. The system gets tested. Minor children, grandparents, aunts and uncles, cousins, even step-relations can experience significant reactions. It is my long-time and hard earned perception of The Family System as " the patient" that brings me to call your attention to this consideration. It's my experience that every family member gets at least a tiny bit of the pathology of trauma. Some overtly display a symptom or two while others suffer in silence. It's more than worth it to stay aware of the possibility, and ask questions if you notice changes that concern you. It is even worth making the suggestion to seek psychotherapy help, to family members who are showing prolonged signs of reactive distress. Don't add to your worry; just stay aware; do your preventative maintenance. Sometimes a really Big System event impacts the relationships Between and Among family members, as well. Big change to any family member affects the whole system. Even really happy changes. Ask the family of any lottery winner.

And now about Chad. Really, i think Chad made the transition to life at the farmhouse quicker and more easily than his Mother or me. He was, of course, younger and more flexible with an abundance of adolescent energy i envied. A saving grace for Chad was his dedicated focus on getting his driver's license. When he acquired a second (or third) hand fixer upper VW, he lived in the driveway totally engaged in his restoration work. When darkness or weather forced him indoors, he was studying for his driver's test or devouring a car part catalog. His fascination with license, car and dating (too soon for me), became a substantial relief for me. At least one aspect of the young man's life was as normal as we could expect.

One unexpected and outstanding benefit of an adolescent getting their license and car is the ripe potential of parental ammunition - made especially sweet if you've been notified, "You're not my real Dad!" Ah......the quintessential conversation of step-parenthood, made even more juicy by being a family therapist and the "Acting" Director of an Adolescent Treatment Facility. More comforting evidence of growing familial normalcy.

It was a delight when Chad took the initiative and secured a retail job once he had his license and a vehicle he had repaired, polished, and accessorized well beyond used car splendor. He also established his own mobile car detailing business - complete with business cards. He had good friends, was well liked for good reason, was getting good grades (thanks, in part, to the threat of restricting access to his vehicle) and was generally making responsible and profitable choices. He was also clever enough and kind enough to protect us from the stuff he knew his Mom and i would have worried over.

Overall, Susan and i agreed on parenting strategies and Chad was considerate and compliant enough to make things work. Although not without the occasional loud protest or an infrequent glass of ice water to supply adequate wakefulness to get to school on time. Again, it was easy to appreciate something else that was going well.

If you are forced to make the radical adjustments a chronic major illness can force upon you, do your best to stay flexible and maintain your sense of humor - it's a genuine asset. Even the most **Serious concerns most often respond better to the softer touch of Sincere.** Personally, i make a conscious effort to respond to "serious" concerns, people, and situations from the far more flexible position of "sincerity".

Being sincere in the face of a serious illness can create enough space to shift your mood. Many times, there's very little chance you can change someone's mind - it's far more useful taking aim at shifting people's mood (for others and yourself).

Small pleasures, a sincere sense of humor, even occasional silliness can offer significant relief (which, with practice, can be amplified into comfort). A case in point from the farmhouse times: admittedly gross Belching Contests. i retired from competition after Chad totally defeated me by belching The Pledge of Allegiance. Now, that's funny - i don't care who you are!

Another cherished activity Chad and i shared was our borderline outrageous grocery shopping trips. i frankly have no idea how we avoided being banned from our local Kroger's. It was at least a couple of years into Susan's recovery toward normalcy before we told her of the raucous nature of our shopping adventures. i worried very little about having to defend my juvenile behavior and clearly poor modeling for impressionable youth as Susan did not care for grocery shopping long before ME/CFS kept her from it. (Shoe shopping was another matter altogether.)

Chad and i bonded over boisterous cruising up and down aisles; him tossing his unbearable adolescent food choices into the cart, me tossing items just as quickly back - sometimes a "no look pass" behind my back or a quick flip backwards over my head. Remember, we were Pros by then. Domesticated shoppers need not apply. To this very day, with he in his forties and i in my early seventies we can become a severe embarrassment to his daughter, Madelyne, (our youngest grandchild). She has threatened to leave the store if we did not, "STOP IT!" and, "Act like grownups!" She was 17 at the time. What can i say? Old habits die hard.

Especially joyful rituals that were at times the only lighthearted moments of freedom from a dreary reality neither of us wanted to share with anyone who was not initiated into the forced life restrictions chronic illness imposes on a family system. So here's the deal: let FUN find you wherever you can; enjoy the relief it brings; appreciate the relief until you feel a soothing effect; amplify the soothing into comfort. Sincerely, that's how humor and laughter heals. Often chronic major illness forces us to make far too many unwanted adjustments. How we make those adjustments is another matter. Focus on what you can get more control over; start with your outlook, your attitudes, your mood. Whenever you can shift from Serious to Sincere. It's a small change AND..........it counts, it matters. You choose.

Thinking back on our time in that old house, i recognize we were often actively working to "make the best" of a crappy bad situation. All three of us have some lovely happy memories of our life there.

i am reminded that Susan first heard a Doctor describing her symptoms on a radio program broadcast by our local PBS affiliate.

i recall how wonderfully strange it was to come home and find her excited and eager to make contact with the Doctor who had a practice treating an illness which fit her symptoms exactly. An illness he referred to as Epstein Barr Virus.

Although he was in an adjoining state, his office was less than two hours away. Doable! She scheduled the appointment from the living room couch that most days she so rightly resented. That appointment was to be a turning point for her, and in true chain reaction form, a happier time for us all. One thing i really hope we did right for Jon and Chad during that time, was to let them know they were loved and valued, no matter how weird their Mother's illness made our lives.

What follows is an account of the exasperations that were too much a part of Susan's first episode with ME/CFS and, sadly, her subsequent relapse eleven years later. The second episode forced her into disability retirement. The discovery that the passage of more than a decade had brought little progress in diagnosis and treatment was troubling enough. Dealing with the widespread ignorance among the medical community at large, AND WORSE, the general lack of curiosity about ME/CFS was often nearly intolerable to me. Susan is a great deal more subtle and civil about this issue than am i. And so, i'm asking you, bear two things in mind as i proceed with this section:

#1 - i do know that what follows is a bit of a "rant". It is not Susan's style to complain - really, she is one of very few humans i've ever met that simply does NOT complain. That seemingly admirable trait can be quite annoying to a practiced complaining whiner such as myself. I do consciously work to limit the, all too male, practice of pouting. Even though i know her to be too classy to offer the sort of report that follows, i'd bet my thumbs she has little disagreement with my account.

#2 - During both episodes, we resolutely fought our way through the brambles and the thickets until we found true Caregiving Gems, our very own Pearls. With persistence we found Physicians, Therapists, Attorneys, Administrators - even Judges - who have proven to be invaluable to Susan being able to cope with this illness. i now have a highly prized list of Professionals who have demonstrated themselves to be caring and compassionate, actively curious, knowledgeable, consistently encouraging, and profoundly competent. The strain of the search has been well worth the find. (What i'm sayin' is, "Don't Give Up!"). There is also now real hope in the recent growth of worldwide coordinated research into ME/CFS. Some of it surprising and most promising. That surge in research is closely related to advocacy efforts aimed at increasing both general knowledge and research funding around ME/CFS. Susan has provided very useful reference sites that i encourage you to explore. There has even been a little progress in getting ME/CFS introduced into Med School Curriculums. (It's just so very unimaginable that it's NOT already standard practice.) Thus begins the Rant.

An unexpected aspect of coping with our new reality in the grasp of ME/CFS was learning to deal with the frequent collisions amid the massive ignorance that then surrounded this illness. Collisions large and small, overt and covert; collisions with the confusion and lack of a reasonable way to understand an illness that could crush you without making you "look sick".

An illness that so often revealed no definitive laboratory results; and major collisions with the established authorities who have the power to make decisions that will profoundly impact your life. We encountered more "authorities" - Physicians, Attorneys, Health Care Administers; of more varieties than i ever imagined existed in our multilayered bureaucratic systems of care. It felt like everyone had forms (nearly always redundant), protocols, and mandatory referrals; while no diagnostic or treatment answers were to be found. Still, the bureaucracy had to be fed.

The most challenging frustration for me as an advocate and family caregiver, was the unexpected ignorance and lack of clinical curiosity among the general medical community. Far far too many physicians when faced with having no reasonable explanation for Susan's admittedly perplexing symptoms, were quick to make a reflexive and grossly inept diagnosis of psychiatric disorders.

We certainly were not out of the norm in experiencing this sort of official response. (That realization would come to light a good bit later as we interacted with other ME/CFS sufferers and their families. Of course, Susan started a support group after recovering enough to get her bearings.) i found the "it must all be in your head" responses so outrageous because Susan and i were family therapists. Both of us were far more familiar with the signs and symptoms of mental disorders than the M.D.'s who simply fell back on psychiatric disorders to explain what they had no other answers for.

The most popular, i was to learn, were Anxiety, Depression or good old fashioned Malingering. i'm frankly surprised some genius didn't exhume the antiquated standbys of Hysteria, Psychoneurotic Disorder, or a serious Conversion Disorder - any one of which could only be approached by years of formal psychoanalysis. (Clearly, i may have some lingering issues from those times.)

In my defense: i was scared, i knew more about mental health problems than they did and, most importantly, i knew Susan. Even when she was profoundly physically weakened, Susan could give me "The Look" that clearly meant, "Honey, just shut up!" when we encountered the "it's all in her pretty little head" response even when it was delivered covertly with sugar coating.

However, sometimes such messages were jarringly overt. Because it feels useful to make a point, i share the following too true story. We had been referred to one of the few "specialists" in CFS in our area at the time of Susan's second episode of ME/CFS. The referral had come from a respected and trusted doctor Susan knew professionally. Because of that referral she received a speedy assessment appointment. The day of the much appreciated expedited appointment, Susan was exceptionally weak and was experiencing significant cognitive and sensory difficulties. If the assessment hadn't been so important we both would have chosen to cancel. Slowly we made the labored trek from the parking lot to the specialist's office. i remember having to fill out the by then all too familiar redundant information form for a new doctor. (This was uncommon for, "I'll do it myself" Susan.)

When we were ushered into the exam room - in slow motion - i had to lift Susan onto the exam table, she was too weak to climb up alone. i then stood beside her so i could steady her and prevent her from falling from the table. It was a scary day. She really needed that assessment.

Upon entering the exam room our specialist seemed to be in a hurry. i'm not certain he even noticed Susan's clear difficulty in breathing. After a quick scan of the paperwork in his hand, that seemed at the very best dismissive, he flatly stated, "I honestly don't even believe in Chronic Fatigue Syndrome". With a clenched jaw, i managed to inquire how he had then become the Specialist in CFS in our area. He lightheartedly related how a Resident whom he was supervising had done a research paper that was fortunate enough to get published. He had signed on to it, as senior team leader. During our 5-10 minute "exam" he took very little notice of Susan. So weakened she was having trouble breathing, Susan, quite uncharacteristically, spoke very little. i assure you, she is more than capable of speaking for herself and i know better than to speak for her under normal circumstances. i do not remember that Doctor touching her during the time he was with us. i am doubtful he even asked any questions.

He certainly wasn't curious enough about the attractive but depleted young woman before him to learn that she had graduated her Master's program Summa Cum Laude, or that she had enjoyed an operative photographic memory, as well as, daily jogging and hiking in the mountains prior to the onset of this illness he didn't even believe in.

My onsite evaluation: this credentialed fool is way too comfortable in his ignorance; while Susan didn't require his competence, she did need his signature. We were face to face with living proof that credentials and competence are not the same thing. It was up to me to get his signature. Thus, i name dropped the physician who referred Susan and how much we had enjoyed his lovely home at a party we had attended there, and how lovely his wife was. The guy was ignorant but thankfully he wasn't stupid. He knew we would report back to the referring doctor. He gave us his hurried signature and his closing summation, "You know, I still don't really believe in Chronic Fatigue Syndrome". Now, that is nuts!

Two quick notes here:
1. *Ignorance is curable by the acquisition of knowledge.*
2. *i managed to refrain from choking the guy with the stethoscope dangling around his neck. My uncommon self restraint, phony smiles and nods along with copious name dropping paid off with him reluctantly signing the form.*

Looking back upon that encounter i deeply appreciate the good fortune of receiving that referral. Susan's professional competence had led to a referral from a highly respected doctor in the State Mental Health System. i'm so thankful he had seen the "Specialist's" name on a published study about CFS. Until i began writing this chapter for Susan, i had tucked that memory away in an appropriately dark corner hoping it might shrivel and croak. However, just now i'm glad it didn't because those kinds of opinions and attitudes are still out there.

If you are in a position of advocacy for a ME/CFS patient, DO NOT ACCEPT THAT KIND OF TREATMENT. Please follow Susan's advice and **Move Away** and **Move On** as soon as possible. We never saw that "Specialist" again, and i never told on him, until now.

How i stayed focused on letting him be right as long as i got my way (his signature on Susan's form) still amazes me. My self restraint probably came from being afraid Susan would fall off the exam table if i removed my arm from her. My point is simply that if you are to be an effective advocate develop fierce resolve, know it can be complicated, confusing and sometimes downright ugly. Stay focused. Keep going. For me the way to deal with the whole "administrative mess" that often surrounds any chronic illness is to focus intensely on whatever piece of the puzzle that needs to be taken care of next. Just do whatever you must to get the next task done. For me, doing what i "must do" required quietly throwing up in my mouth, with fake smiles and nods.

Still, Persist. It's worth it. When the dust clears, you will be rewarded by finding compassionate, competent, professional caregivers that will likely become some of your favorite humans. At least it has gone that way for me.

One final thought about being an effective advocate. You will need to find a way to care for yourself. You simply can't give your best if you're not at your best. For me that meant allowing family to support and nurture Me. It also meant finding the humor that lurks in strange places - sometimes dark and even sick humor. But, "Hey!", a laugh is a laugh. Laughter is therapeutic and healing - look it up. Music was also a refuge for me, both listening and playing. i was blessed with an alto saxophone in the 5th grade and i've been making noise ever since. If there is some activity that has brought you pleasure, keep it as active in your life as you can. i also found keeping a journal to vent my frustrations about the "rat bastards" i wasn't allowed to choke or the tears i somehow choked back, was a genuinely useful tool. i also recommend a separate Appreciation Journal where you remind yourself of all the things that touch your life daily, that really make the struggle worth it. Start with three things a day: like an interesting shaped cloud, a taste of ripe orange, a comfy pillow - you get the idea. Make a habit of noticing little things that soothe you, bring you relief, sustain you. Notice nice things on purpose.

On the downside i recognize now that i fell into a less than optimal pattern of compensatory eating - overeating. It was a family pattern from my childhood. i had been domesticated at a very young age to believe that there was no injury, physical or emotional, that eating wouldn't soothe. My Grandma could stop the flow of blood from an open wound by giving you a couple of her deliciously warm oatmeal raisin cookies. But overeating was a better choice than alcohol or drugs or gambling or any number of other life injuring vices. Looking back, regular exercise, yoga, meditation or (make your own list that fits your interest) would have been better choices. i encourage you to intentionally Decide that it's not just OK to take care of yourself, it is honestly necessary.

Be at your Best to give the ones you love, your Best. Know that you likely won't win every battle. You may often fall short - go figure. At the end of many challenging and frustrating days of dealing with ME/ CFS your refuge and peace of mind rests in knowing that you did your best; and, you are not going to give up. Do your best. Don't quit. Keep your Sense of Humor. Limit the oatmeal raisin cookies. You Got This!

Speaking of doing your best brings me back to my amazing Susan. One of the many traits i admire and love about Susan is that she not only always (but in all ways) does her personal best, and she is also annoyingly dedicated to doing all (and i mean everything) she can do each and every day, in pretty much every way. She doesn't think in terms of a day-or-two off. Now you might wonder how always doing all you can, could be annoying. Well, she continues to live with ME/ CFS; AND, one of the most practical and productive strategies we have discovered is to strategically REST FORWARD.

My monitoring of her energy expenditures is probably my most irritating behavior for her. That's saying quite a bit in light of my many peculiarities. "Better slow down Dear." "This might be the perfect time to Rest Forward." Or the more crass admonishments of, "Please! Stop Now!" "Honey really; check yourself before you wreck yourself." "Do you know you've been working over an hour and a half with- out a break?" Well, of course she knows - most of the time. i have learned to lean away from asking, "Sweetie, why don't you at least just sit down with me for a few minutes?" i don't ask that anymore because i've learned the answer, "Michael, if I sit down now I'm afraid I won't be able to get back up". And that's the difficult truth.

That she just won't quit is difficult because it is both a Blessing and a Curse. Over the many years of living with this illness, her abso- lute commitment to doing her very best, to doing the most she can, working (spending precious energy) until whatever she's focused on gets done - or at least the chunk she had set for her goal that day - has been her consistent hallmark. Clearly a Blessing [but, a cursed blessing]. Remember, a major defining aspect of ME/CFS is PEM - Post Exertion Malaise. [Please know how fed up i am with all the new capital lettered initials this illness has dragged into my awareness. All those acronyms have become about as welcome as the dead rodents and rabbits our much loved cat would leave on our doorstep back at the farmhouse.] PEM is really about your bounce back time, the amount of time it takes to recover from exertion - whether that exertion be physical or mental or emotional. The greater the exertion, the longer the recovery time, has proven to be a realistic expectation. i often need to remind myself how huge an imposition that constraint is to a life-long overachiever, a maker of endless (and practical) lists, a dedicated and highly skilled goal setter who knows the specifics of establishing well formed outcomes. That's our Susan. She knows what she wants and she makes a plan to get it (goals, Goals, GOALS!).

"Better slow down Dear." she don't do well with; especially when she knows my unspoken worried thought is, "i'm just so afraid you'll pay for overworking with a couple of days in bed; or worse, BabyGirl, with a horrible major relapse episode". Who the heck needs to hear that while they are doing exactly what has been the greatest single asset in dealing with this illness. Certainly not my fierce Susan.

Being realistic about her expenditure of energy is a daily issue. Decisions about our schedule and planned activities are frequently con-flicted. Being realistic without underachieving or, perhaps worse, under expecting can feel dangerously close to acquiescence. Any thought of giving up is not an option! i told you, she is fierce. "Overdoing it" has punishing PEM consequences that have proven non-negotiable. That is why finding a balance is crucial. Why Resting Forward is a productive and valuable choice. Finding that balance is why we bump heads from time to time. That head bumping might leave less lumps if we both weren't so certain that we know everything and that we both believe we know best. Bumps? Sure - but "Love Bumps".

A bit more that is useful to know about (my) Susan. She is not only real smart, capable, creative, determined (to a fault), ethical, compas-sionate, generous, loyal, (there's more but she will certainly edit it out if i truthfully gush further) but also effortlessly glamorous. She is one of those rare people who can come in from doing yard work in her muddy "grunges" and look like she just walked off a Hollywood movie set. i swear. Her style is legendary among those who know her and look to her for her impeccable style and exemplary good taste. i have often told her of my perception that she doesn't wear clothes, only costumes.

i often have the feeling people who see us together must think she is walking her strange two legged dog. We are a somewhat confusing (but not conflicted) combination of classy and crude (but cute-ish).

After Susan fought her way back from her initial episode of utter collapse with ME/CFS - an arduous journey of very nearly three years - she was determined to realize her goal of returning to full time (and properly compensated) employment. She secured the position of Assistant Director of Social Work at the two Psychiatric Hospitals in our area. They were quick to recognize the qualities (and more) that i've described and promoted her to the duties of Forensic Liaison, responsible for dealing with patients with criminal court involvement and eventually, Clinical Care Coordinator. Both positions required her attention and presence at both locations on occasion. Both locations were about a 2 hour drive from one another. One was 45 minutes from our home, the other an hour and a half. Travel time was an issue when 10 hour days were the norm. She was back "full time" and then some.

Being Forensic Liaison meant routinely interacting with Judges and court systems in 17 counties served by the two hospitals. This number expanded to 20 counties with the closure of another local psychiatric hospital. More road time. On several occasions she was even responsible for interaction with the FBI and CIA in patient related forensic matters.

And still that wasn't enough stress and responsibility for Susan. She also established active and well attended Family Support Groups at both facilities. On weekends, of course, because that's when families can attend. She wasn't about to neglect her family therapy roots - even when it meant driving to both hospitals one weekend a month. Susan is the kind of leader that models what she expects of those she leads. The Family Support Groups were an unquestionable success and were deeply valued by patients, as well as families. Staff at both hospitals were overwhelmingly positive in their support and active participants in those Group Weekends. i know. i was there for a bunch of them.

After about six years in this rewarding and challenging position, an even more challenging position in the State Department of Mental

Health became open: Area Director for the State Department of Mental Health - there were only six Area Directors in the State System. Of course, she applied. Of course, she got the job. Of course, she chose to serve the 20 county area that was geographically largest and demographically smallest of all six areas.

Add to the challenges the daunting task of advocating for equal funding for the poorest counties with the least votes in the state. Add the expectation of navigating state politics to your job duties. She was now responsible for overseeing and guiding the administration of outpatient community mental health services and coordinating with State Department Psychiatric Hospital Administration for all inpatient services in 20 counties. Oh, and of course, the rotating occasional weekend 24 hour on call duty of managing high profile statewide mental health emergencies, alerting necessary parties of incidents and arranging emergency assistance for all who needed help. (i remember one such incident of a fire in a mental health group home.)

The State Department recognized her success in her position at the hospitals and her excellent performance in her Area Director position, and sent her to a post graduate Executive Leadership Program at Case Western Reserve University, a semester timeframe of every other week Friday treks to Cleveland - even more road time to accommodate into her schedule. Susan also represented the State Mental Health Department on national projects that had her traveling from Baltimore, Maryland for a Schizophrenia Research Study to Portland, Oregon for National Rural Mental Health Studies. After several years of being essentially home bound (many days bed bound), now Susan was only home to sleep, too little (after a quick convenient meal); then she was routinely leaving before sun-up to attend appointments throughout the 20 counties she served. Susan insisted on getting out of her State Capitol Office where many small, poor counties were financially pressed to attend meetings - and held meetings in the many communities for which she was responsible. A change in normal state protocol, but approved wholeheartedly by State Mental Health Administration in supporting Susan's area known for it's poverty. All that travel allowed her to really get to know the populations and cultures she worked so hard to serve.

My forty minute commute (one way) to and from my work was annoying enough - but completely insignificant by comparison.

i report all of this - which Susan will most certainly want to omit (i've never heard her brag, her parents would never have permitted it and i'm certain she simply views what i see as significant and praiseworthy achievements as simply doing her job). i'm telling all this "good stuff" about her to say this: one of the most astounding things i have repeatedly heard her say during her ongoing battle with ME/CFS is, "I just feel so lazy ". Susan does not do lazy.

i could tutor her in "lazy". i'm the one slouched on the couch in front of T.V. saying, "Sweetheart, could you reach over there and hand me the remote. Oh yeah.....Please." When she says she feels lazy i've learned that it's her ME/CFS speak for, "My dearest Wonder Spouse Michael, today I am so profoundly exhausted that it is an effort to just blink, let alone think. If I weren't so viciously tired I fear I would be dangerously angry to the point of hateful about this miserable crap! But just this red hot minute, I don't have the energy for it." Yes. i am a very fluid translator of ME/CFS speak. You're Welcome.

The point of this embarrassing (to Susan) report is this: The people who become afflicted with ME/CFS are too often seen as malingering and/or "lazy" - because they don't particularly "look sick". At least at first fleeting glance. If you were to look more closely through better informed eyes you would notice moderately to severely impaired breathing, that is often uncommonly shallow. You could also see a pale pallid countenance - always disguised by perfect subtle makeup when we were in public, at appointments, or even at family social events. If you were to listen with better educated ears, you would hear an uncommonly soft volume in speaking voice. It's quite difficult to produce a robust tone of voice when the muscles that operate the physical mechanisms of breath and speech are just too fatigued to do their job adequately. With Susan, i can hear a distinctive telltale vocal timbre, a subtle rasp, that reliably alerts me to a low energy day - even when i hear it over the phone. There are also clear indicators in both posture and gait. Poker players call these signs "tells"; and they're willing to bet big on them. In my NLP (Neuro Linguistic Programming) Training, systemically seeing and hearing those "tells" was given the name "calibration skills". My point is, be willing to look and listen more deeply to loved ones with ME/CFS.

Let me be unapologetically clear, telling someone with ME/CFS, "Well you sure don't look sick." will hardly ever be taken as a compliment. It is more likely to be taken as an insulting insinuation that, "You're Not Really sick". Or, "You're fakin' it". So just don't say that unless, of course, you are for some strange reason determined to demonstrate your ignorance and gross insensitivity. It is my hope that you find this hint helpful if you're new to ME/CFS; i'm certain folks struggling with it will.

Consider further, what seems to me a tragic misnaming of this illness. First dubbed the dismissive "Yuppie Flu". Then upgraded to Epstein Barr Virus and then to CFS (Chronic Fatigue Syndrome). Chronic fatigue conveys "being tired a bunch". "Everybody gets tired don't they? People who get tired a bunch are probably really out of shape or just lazy, and certainly too lazy to exercise their way back to strength. Chronic fatigue, my bottom! Why not just declare laziness an official disease?"

And then there's the Syndrome part - "Ain't that just like a tiny little baby disease?" Well actually, "No". A Syndrome can kill you just as dead as a Disease. The only difference is a lab test. True. True. True. A single lab test, when found, will end CF**S**. The Syndrome will be a historic artifact.

More recently, the name SEID (Systemic Exertion Intolerance Disorder) was more appropriately suggested but didn't capture clearly enough the varied and profound neurological and sensory symptoms of what will some day soon i pray, make it to the elite status of disease. Hopefully simultaneously with effective treatment, if not an outright cure. ME (Myalgic Encephalomyelitis) captures the neurological significance but i would personally like it, for simple accuracy - if the official name spoke to Post Exertion Malaise; SEID seems far closer to calling it what it is than Chronic Fatigue.

The point of this mini rant? Be aware of how much harm adding ignorant and outright inconsiderate comments can bring. One of the truly important things you **CAN** do as a support person or family member of a ME/CFS sufferer is to get informed. Convincingly, let the people you care for KNOW THAT YOU BELIEVE THEM. Let them know that you Know they are not simply being lazy or pretending to be ill. Consistently let them know through the multiple, often shifting, curious, sometimes downright mysterious and seemingly endlessly evolving and most baffling symptoms of this "not quite yet" disease, that you are there with them and for them. And always, in all ways, in every way you can, let them know you Believe them. It won't cure it; but i promise; it'll make a comforting difference.

THE SEX STUFF!

So guys (and gals too, if your partner is dealing with the life limiting impositions ME/CFS presents), now is as good a time as any to have "THE TALK". The S-E-X talk.

[Jon, Chad, and Growed Up Grandkids: Yes! i certainly am going to discuss this *touchy* and often embarrassing topic. How unlike me. Deal with it.]

Now Sex. We sincerely need to talk about sex with ME/CFS or, more specifically, what can very quickly become a serious issue - the absence of sex with ME/CFS. i know it sounds cray - cray, but when you feel like you're fighting off the worst flu you can remember - and losing that fight, when you ache all over - and all under, when your skin is so sensitive to the touch even the finest flannel sheets are feeling scratchy, when soft lights are way too bright and direct sunlight hurts, when just a whisper is too loud and normal sound levels feel like illegal auditory assault, when you can't really tell if you're more sick or you're more tired; when you are so sick and so tired you quite literally can not think straight, when you're having scary unexplained memory blips, when you can't read because you can't recall what you read two sentences ago, let alone the two preceding paragraphs; well, there's a pretty fair chance you won't be feeling all that horny. "All right. All right, Susan! Amorous." There are times with ME/CFS if the hottest heartthrob you could conjure were to bat their flirty-flirty eyes at you, the sexual impulse that you wish you had just would not override the YUK. There it is. The nutshell, elevator pitch version of the ME/CFS sex talk. But wait, there's more (at least i ain't done yet).

If you are the one struggling with ME/CFS every hour of every day, you could simply refuse to accept any and all mention of sex. This may be accomplished overtly, "Oh, Hell No!" or covertly, "Oh, that's so sweet of you to ask, maybe later. (Yeah! Really Really Later)".

Either way, you will almost certainly get to add disappointment, frustration, guilt - perhaps to the point of shame, and a case of worry (that's batting its flirty eyes at some nasty ongoing anxiety) to your already overloaded daily burden. Of course, you could choose to be totally phony and pretend to be "amorous" and just comply with every request for sex you could tolerate. The downside of that choice is steadily growing resentment and eventual alienation from a person you, once upon a time, loved being loving with; and then you're paving the path to self-loathing. (Also, when you "pretend" and go-along-to-get-along, just to "shut 'em up", even the most ardent of partners will catch on and feel disappointed and dissatisfied.). Now, if you are the partner bold enough to make a "likely to be rejected" sexual approach, you have to get familiar with feeling at risk, with knowing your well intentioned loving request is almost certainly going to be received as an unwanted imposition. And get prepared to deal with resentment if you are rebuffed, denied, deprived of what's rightfully yours. [If you feel this way, you are most certainly a guy - regardless of your gender.] And if you are reluctantly or insincerely granted your request, get ready to feel a nagging guilt and sense of disappointment - in both your partner and yourself.

i'm just sayin', sex or no sex with ME/CFS often (nearly always) gets tricky. It can become a very real extra burden, the "adding insult to injury" kind - for both partners. And, again, nearly always, being too confused, embarrassed or just plain afraid to talk about it, makes it worse. The silence of unspeakability amplifies the problem far more often than it helps. Thus, i suggest finding a way to talk about it. And since the SEX parts can become so quickly inflamed (i couldn't resist...not even sorry....lighten up), allow me to suggest we start by thinking about *Intimacy*. After all, the really "good sex" always has intimacy for its roommate.

Certainly, there is no argument that intimacy and sex are the most attractive of bed partners. That being an undisputed fact, certainly to me, i want to be clear that sex and intimacy can and do occur separately - far too often. In some physically healthy but emotionally wounded relationships, they live in completely different zip codes.

It's a well known fact that "the sex thing" in relationships with no health challenges to interfere at all, is Big Business. In the U.S., the red hot demand for sex help is filling the shelves of booksellers with an ever expanding selection. Sex, or the dysfunction there of, has made Dr. Phil - and Dr. Ruth before him - richer than they might have dared dream. Sex Therapy is a thriving enterprise in a culture that sells everything from toothpaste to clothing to vacation rentals and the sexy automobiles that get you there with heavy doses of **S!E!X!** And still, so many of us can't talk about [it.]

In years of dealing professionally with couples who were both quite physically healthy, the root problem was, far too often, sex had stayed in their house while intimacy had moved away - quite a while before the couple had made their way to my office. The vast majority of those couples couldn't find their way to talking about sex on their own. All too often the painful reality was far too many reluctant partners only agreed to come to a therapy session so they could drop their unwanted spouse/partner off for some unsuspecting do-gooder therapist to take care of - like leaving an unwanted rescue dog dropped off on someone's doorstep in the dead of night. Clearly, they waited way too long to talk about "It". My professional experience informs me that sex with no real intimacy makes for a troublesome prognosis in therapy. The sex stuff is comparatively easier to repair when intimacy is still alive - even if it's on life support.

It is also worth noting the couples whose relationship ended not because one of the partners was sexually "unfaithful"; rather it was because they did something far more hurtful and harder to forgive - they committed emotional intimacy outside the bounds and bonds of their relationship. Intimacy. Sex. Each can exist without the other. But the real beating heart of the matter is INTIMACY.

If ME/CFS has imposed itself on the sexual intimacy in your relationship, it's really no surprise at all. If it has NOT become an obstacle,

That is truly remarkable. Noteworthy, in fact, and deserving of close study. This strange illness will test all your relationships: sexual, social, familial, financial, cultural and maybe most profoundly your intra-personal relationship within yourself.

i think the test presented intra-personally may be the most difficult of all, because it is so subtle and again, too seldom mentioned. All that to say, with ME/CFS you can expect SEX to be different. Maybe radically different. Perhaps entirely absent for periods. The good news is, Intimacy can thrive even without sexy-sexy.

Having the "sex talk" for couples dealing with ME/CFS is so vital because it opens a door into the place where loving tender intimacy resides. When you allow the topic of sex to remain unspeakable, you give it far more power than it deserves. Years ago i wrote the poem below that came to mind as i was writing this segment of the seemingly endless "chapter" Susan requested. (So, "Yes". i am blaming my long-windedness on her.) The Poem:

<blockquote>
Distance is in the
I
Of the Withholder.
</blockquote>

Staying silent about sex when you both know it is a real problem qualifies as willful lying, a sin of OMISSION, a Big Mistake - at least by my reckoning. Staying silent about sex invites growing resentment and misunderstanding. If you are suffering with ME/CFS and are thinking your partner SHOULD KNOW that you are sick, too sick for sex; If you are thinking they SHOULD KNOW BETTER than to take your lack of interest in sex personally: YOU ARE WAY WRONG! "Yes", you can be sick and tired AND wrong. "Yes", having the sex talk is going to ZAP your energy in all likelihood. And "Yes!" dealing directly with the problem could help preserve your relationship. Your partner may not be the gifted psychic you wish for - especially if your partner is a "guy" who has been culturally domesticated to believe that INTIMACY = SEX. Investing energy in "The sex talk" can pay huge dividends for you and your partner; but perhaps most importantly, for your RELATIONSHIP. The sex talk is for the Relationship most of all.

Next, i feel it is useful to make clear what i mean by INTIMACY. This feels necessary because our society has too often downgraded intimacy solely to the context of SEXUAL intimacy.

i am asking the reader to consider a broader and yet more focused view of intimacy, where sex can be absent or present. Intimacy is the core focus. Here i define intimacy as being an essential part of an affectionate and loving personal relationship. i am speaking of an intimacy built upon a foundation of loving appreciation of the other (AND the SELF) - a comfortable and comforting warm familiarity that is deeper and much more durable than sex. Intimacy that has trust and loyal friendship at its root. The intimacy i speak of here is born of compassion, not pity.

The intimacy i advocate here lasts far longer than even the best sex. And, yes, deep intimacy is probably, in the end, the sexiest thing on earth! BUT/AND THE PROBLEM HERE IS: folks with ME/CFS just ain't feelin' the sex thing - even when they desperately wish they were! AND STILL, as sick and as tired as they may be, they can receive real relief, soothing and comfort from expressions of intimacy offered from a loving partner who knows to offer that intimacy with no demands for or expectation of sex.

The kind of intimacy i'm speaking of is often found in a cherished childhood friendship, in the private intimate relationship with a beloved pet, with your closest sibling, perhaps with someone you served with in the military, or with an old teammate whose friendship naturally continued beyond the games played in childhood. That sort of intimacy can not only be kept alive but can keep growing with no sex whatsoever. The intimacy i am encouraging can be a relationship saver when illness prevents normal healthy sexuality.

It is my sincere and SERIOUS hope that i have made clear how strongly i believe it is essential to break the Silence Barrier and make sex speakable in your relationship. With or without ME/CFS.

You can expect it to be uncomfortable. And you can expect it to be of greater value than you imagined.

I also hope i have clarified my idea of the kind of intimacy that can support, nurture and even save a relationship. And here's a thought about both "the sex talk" and "intimacy - non sexual style".

LOVE NOTES: Write each other Love Notes about what you wish you could say, about what you wish you knew, about how you are feeling, about what you are afraid of, and/ or about your hopes for your relationships. Maybe you kids will surprise yourselves. Of course that's risky. Yet, staying silent is a lot more risky. (And, oh yeah, if you decide to try the Love Notes - buy some special stationery - it'll give the experiment some extra momentum.)

All that to say this: STAY IN TOUCH with your partner whether you are in the role of sufferer or supporter. There is a wealth of research data about how loving human touch affects us. *(And i do realize there are sad exceptions where "being touched" is anchored to traumatic memories that have been unwittingly carried into present moment circumstances. And please remember that i also believe in the absolute possibility of successful treatment of those traumatic memories. But that's a whole book by itself. Another time maybe.)* It is my strong personal and professional opinion that you should Not neglect Touch. Maintain physical contact in your relationship. Making touching taboo doesn't just "add insult to injury", i believe it adds "more injury to the existing injury". Hugs, kissing, cuddling, handholding (even in public), foot massages, and shoulder rubs can affirm and amplify NON-SEXUAL intimacy. (Remember, be gentle. So many folks with ME/CFS have a coexisting diagnosis of Fibromyalgia which often presents with bunches of physical pain.) Susan and i have found Reiki to be an an alternative that can provide both relief and comfort, and can enhance our mutual feelings of intimacy. Maintaining affectionate non-sexual physical contact is more than important, it is essential. So, STAY IN TOUCH - if you're thinking intimacy might be worth the effort in your relationship.

And again guys - yes, almost always guys - pay close attention to the signs and signals you are getting from your partner during a happy foot massage. i remind you to pay attention because even in spite of your good intentions to keep sex out of the way, if you're healthy you're likely to feel a little horny - maybe a lot. You have been domesticated to get confused from "Boys will be Boys" rolling around in your head onward toward adulthood. (i am fairly sure i gotta whole book on "Boys will be Boys" rolling around in my head.)

In our culture like many others, men are programmed to be overly aggressive sexually and to feel equally overly privileged to do so. i'm sayin' that's not simply my opinion; it's solid Social Science. If you care about intimacy beyond sex, pay attention. Even ask your partner for a "Safe Word" if you find it too tough to read the response you're getting. i'm really not trying to stir up trouble; i'm trying to keep a sweet thing from going sour. By the way, when you learn how to nurture your intimacy with non-sexual physical contact, getting back to the sex stuff, when energy and comfort allows, is so much easier.

So, if you are doing your best to give an honestly innocent shoulder rub and you hear your partner say, "Ah, that feels nice.", it almost certainly Does Not mean, "Ah Yeah Baby! Bring it on Big Guy! Your magic touch has cured ME/CFS!! Let's Get It On!!!". It is far more likely that, "Ah, that feels nice." means that it feels nice. That feels nice, as in: "That helped take my mind off all the bills I am worried I will never get paid" or, "That's the first I have felt relaxed all week" or, "I'm finally thinking you may still care for me when I feel helpless and useless" or simply just, "Thank you for understanding". i'm trying to encourage you to move beyond the normal "guy" response - even if you're a gal. The kind of touch i hope to address is about caring, compassion and emotional connection - about reassurance; then maybe when you hear, "Ah, that's nice". You can mean it when you respond, "Yeah, it really is nice".

You can often find real and comforting intimacy in sharing activities you both enjoy. Movies can become opportunities to share your unique viewpoints on story and movie craft. You can listen to music together and share your thoughts. You might even take a chance on a slow dance. Attending a lecture at your public library or nearby college offers a chance to listen to your partner's perception. Learning how a person you truly care for views the world is very intimate indeed. Books, paintings, concerts all offer us a chance to get curious about, listen to and learn from one another. We have found exploring Netflix to be a very valuable option when it's just too tired to get dressed and leave the house. You're allowed to make a "couch date" and plan to listen to each other's reaction and opinion about what you've just experienced together. Plan to be curious about your partners experience. You, as a couple, are allowed to intentionally commit the intimacy that the sex stuff may have been blocking. You know, Emotional Intimacy.

You might think that's all about that. But, "Oh No". i go on, because misunderstanding a lack of interest in things sexy-sexy, and taking it as a Personal Rejection is a disturbingly common Mistake. A really major Mistake. Think about it. Even if you are in a advanced state of "amorous arousal", you just might lose all interest in Hubba-Hubba when the car in your garage explodes into flames and knocks down a wall or two. Your focus changes radically when you're under threat. So guys - of all genders and orientations - slow your roll. Don't be too quick to take it personally. It almost certainly is NOT about YOU. It's most likely a simple energy shortage. Like when you discover the gas tank in your mower is empty, and the gas can is bone dry, AND you really really wanted to cut the grass - it needed done, it was way overdue, urgent! Do you complain and whine and pout? Sure. We all do. But it's clearly a good time to pause and make a plan to refuel.

Now, i am aware there are those who would remind me that all of this understanding, romance and intimacy stuff is fine, BUT sex is a basic need for everyone - like air and food and water! And i will point out: you don't expect your partner to take your next breath for you, and you can certainly take a bite of a juicy Wally Burger and chew it all by yourself, and you long ago mastered swallowing a refreshing gulp of water without the help of another. In the unlikely case you have not caught the drift of this latest mini rant; i'll review: breathing, eating, drinking can all be accomplished without assistance. And sex? i'm fairly certain you can handle that too.

Far too many humans have been influenced to judge how much they are loved by how much sex they are currently getting, humans of both genders and all orientations. i believe "frequency of sex" to be a flawed, misleading, and detrimental measure of how much we are loved - especially when it is the only metric being considered. Real intimacy is both a far better choice and measuring principle.

Further, i would like to offer some thoughts about how to promote a mood of intimacy within ourselves. One of the most practical and powerful things we can do to invite intimacy into our lives in general is to focus our attention on Appreciation. Intentionally focus on Actively Appreciating things large and small. Take notice of a friendly smile (received or given), a happy bird's song, real friends, sunny skies, even an unexpected great parking spot. DECIDE to appreciate with focused intent. You could even carry an inexpensive little note pad to jot down appreciations so you could enjoy them later, quietly on purpose, or even transcribe them into an Appreciation Journal. Why Appreciation? Because the frequency of Appreciation is so near the vibrations of Compassion and Love. And that's about as intimate as any of us can get. Appreciate with focused intent on Music, Art, Loyalty, Freedom, your Pets, Friends. A simple thing i appreciate more deeply than i can explain is the sound of our beloved dog lapping water from her bowl.

Once you can get yourself focused into a general mood of Appreciation, you are better prepared to explore and expand intimacy with your partner. Again, Appreciation is only a blink and a breath away from Love. Approaching your partner with deep and Loving Appreciation generates nearly effortless intimacy. When your frame of reference is mutual appreciation of one another, honest communication is far easier. Maybe even the "sex talk" will get easier.

If you're doing your best to discuss sex or any other troublesome issues in your relationship, and you find it just too difficult and you arrive at an impasse - hire a good plumber right away. Wait, did i say plumber? Plumbers are for plugged up non-functioning toilets (which are pretty important to a happy home). Really, if you find yourselves stuck Do Not let your emotional toilets backup; they will eventually overflow and you will have an even bigger mess. Of course, i suggest you try a Therapist, Counselor, or Minister. Often the particular person you hire is far less important than the fact that you have both come to the agreement that seeking help really is that important. And should it prove too difficult or expensive to find a professional to help clear your metaphorical clog, you could go buy almost any sex self-help book. The specific book you select is way less important than the act of reading and discussing that book As A Couple. The trick to making it work for you is to aim your comments at "the Book". That way you avoid disagreeing with your partner. Stick to sharing your responses and opinions of the Book. If you can manage to be genuinely curious about your partner's viewpoint and opinions, you will have managed to have a discussion about a topic that was formerly unspeakable. Now that's progress.

Does ME/ CFS force concessions on your relationship? Most certainly; often major ones. Are major concessions worth the effort? Is the preservation of commitment and dedication, and the deep satisfaction those qualities bring to your life, worth the adjustments that are demanded? This is a most serious question. A question only you can ask yourself.

Here is a happy truth that no chronic debilitating illness can change: It Is Never Too Late, Or Too Soon, To Experience Emotional Growth. i have twisted that line from a quote by perhaps my favorite author, Tom Robbins, who penned it this way, "It's never too late to have a happy childhood". This is Earth, after all, where "CONTRAST HAPPENS" - to paraphrase a more coarse bumper sticker. For certain, the only thing that doesn't change throughout our lives is that change is coming. Change is the constant common factor in all our lives. Knowing that inescapable certainty, try viewing Obstacles ME/CFS places in your path as curious Opportunities. That is, after you catch your breath from kicking and screaming and stamping out your frustrations at those unwanted changes. It really is possible to view the undeniably difficult issues surrounding sex with ME/CFS as an opportunity to look inward, in order to discover what intimacy means to you. You may just find being determined to fight your way through all the ME/

CFS crap together as partners can fertilize deep and satisfying new growth - both as a couple and individually.

You will, at least from time to time, be either forced to or asked to choose between Intimacy and Sex. Sex does offer quick and pleasurable satisfaction (if you can keep guilt and disappointment out of the bedchamber). Intimacy brings real lasting affection, ever deepening appreciation, enduring friendship, loyalty, perhaps even mutual admiration, and spiritual connection, and, well.............., Love actually.

And that, actually, feels pretty sexy-sexy to me.

So now where was i.......

We have certainly had our share of dark days and disappointments where Susan's characteristic optimism was dampened - even close to dormant. Perhaps one of the greatest challenges she has faced was being forced into disability retirement from her position at the State Department of Mental Health. She had clear GOALS and detailed plans to achieve them. She cared, still cares, passionately about serving people by improving the system of care. i became acutely aware that the loss of your professional self, a critical element of your sense of self, was in fact and in deed, a palpable reality. A crushing loss and yet another thing about which to be deeply sickened.

Most people (certainly myself included) would cry and cry until all the tears dried up. i helplessly looked on while Susan did her share of that complete with the very understandable, even expected, reactive agitated depression. But when she caught her breath, she fell back on her core values and instincts - she got busy and set new goals aimed at doing what she could. And all the way doing her best everyday, regardless of how strong or how weak her best was from day to day. To my stunned amazement and complete admiration, she started a home based business. Not one but two. The first business was SWEET TREATS. Susan applied for and received a license through the Federal Department of Agriculture and had our kitchen approved to bake and sell succulent gourmet chocolate chip cookies. She used the best ingredients to produce oversized "show cookies". She used her version of a recipe that had an allegedly murky history. They were labor intensive and required that you grind your own whole oats to ensure the "right" taste and texture. With Susan there certainly was a "right way". The cookies were extra large with both dark chocolate chips and dark chocolate chunks. Once baked, she inserted long stem like sticks and gift wrapped them carefully, elaborately in red translucent cellophane and adorned them with handmade bows - of the just right ribbon. Those sweet babies were then arranged like fancy flower arrangements in a vase or long stem rose box or any reasonable request for custom presentation. Those cookies were "the Bomb". They always received rave reviews. Those cookies were way too much trouble for most folks to make themselves. Those cookies made a statement - they really were Sweet Treats.

While i more than once wondered if they were worth the effort, i also recognized that Susan could plan ahead to produce an order and she could work in intervals that matched her available energy. This often meant working for 15 minutes and then having to rest for half an hour; on and off in that pattern until she finished an order.

i got to help in the grunt work, grocery shopping and the occasional delivery. (i fondly recall squeals of joy when recipients would first lay eyes on Susan's impressive creations.) Even though producing a batch was almost always a major chore, she planned every batch for overproduction due to insistent family demand. (Sorry Grandma, your cookies couldn't compete with these - yeah, that good!)

i wanted to tell this true story because it demonstrates Susan's persistence, style and uncanny ability to turn "Yuk" into "Yum".

Another business Susan conceived and operated from home was Hole' Mole' (pronounced *Holy Moly*) Creations. Oh yeah, she sews too - and beautifully. i still wear the hats and scarves she created for me. She has sent Poodle Skirts all over the U.S. and several times across the Atlantic. (This sprang from a request by our oldest granddaughter, Kelsey, wanting a poodle skirt to wear to her school dance.) Susan too seldom wears some of the very fetching pieces she has designed, but when she does, she never fails to receive compliments and questions about, "Where did you find this?". She had created another home business that allowed her to work at her own on and off ME/CFS dictated pace. One of my favorite items she came up with were one-of-a-kind-fancy-schmancy wine bags which she successfully marketed to several upscale wine shops in our area. Those bags could turn the cheapest bottle into a very attractive gift. She even tried marketing her original fashion designs, unique purses, and wine bags at several Art and Craft Festivals. Being a vendor proved too taxing with the long hours and stress of dealing with the patrons and other vendors at shows. So of course, she adjusted. She downsized to online sales.

To this day Susan is the "go to" seamstress for family. Any needed alterations to prom gowns, bride's maid dresses, even several wedding gowns, our granddaughter, Siena's, have received Susan's capable and elegant touch. And of course, i would not think of insulting her by taking any of my alterations or mending needs to anyone else.

i have yet to mention the Home and Garden worthy landscaping Susan has created around our home. People have actually stopped while driving by to take pictures and offer compliments (which i most graciously accept). Many days she gets up by sunrise and works in 15 - 30 minute bursts before the temperature and/or humidity becomes too great (another thing that was never an issue before ME/CFS). She then often returns in the hours before sunset to do a little more, if able. Little by little, day after day, doing however much that day's energy permitted, she has created a landscape of remarkable beauty. Really, i've got the photos to prove it. It's taken a number of years but that's not much of an obstacle if you know you're never going to quit. The point of telling this? Susan does a whole lot for a woman who reports feeling "lazy". Sure, her and Wonder Woman. The way i see it, she is Wonder Woman.

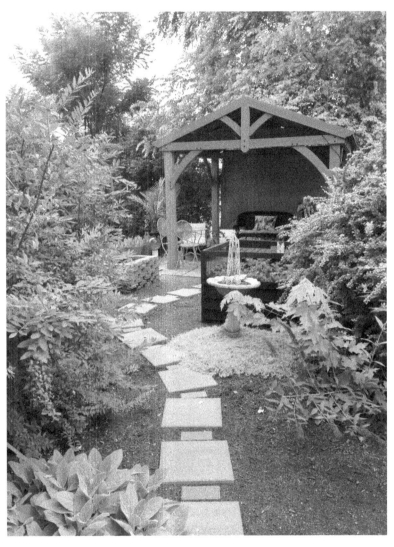

Susan started this project in 2003 when all she could manage was to work for a maximum of ten to fifteen minutes at a time. She would plant a few flowers and pull a few weeds, and she was happy. Each year she added few flowers and she slowly began to build paths as she was able. In 2017 we decided to have our niece's husband construct this pavilion so we could staycation with ME/CFS. In 2018 she was only able to work in the yard three times the entire summer. In 2019 she worked early mornings with little to no relapse, so she was able to accomplish more in the gardens, but her main accomplishment was pure happiness.

Right now she is formatting the final draft of this book. It will be ready to send to the publishers after my tardy contribution is completed. Yesterday she informed me she had worked out the concept and rough outline for her next book. i am often in the position where i'm uncertain whether i want to scream or cheer. "Honey, you might consider slowing down and just take it easy." (Not really likely - just ain't gonna happen.)

i would be remiss if i did not speak about Susan's commitment to advocacy for ME/CFS research funding. i encourage you to review Susan's excellent letter to our Senators at the end of this book, and feel free to use it as a format for your own advocacy efforts. We have found that letters and phone calls are logged and reported to your elected officials. They are working for you. ME/CFS is not only largely misunderstood, it is also a major worldwide healthcare crisis. ME/CFS is still massively underfunded in the United States. Your calls and letters to politicians have a positive impact. Your voice truly matters. You really can help your elected representatives serve you better.

A couple of years ago, we made a pilgrimage to Washington, D.C. for the Second Annual "Solve ME Advocacy" event. Solve ME had prearranged appointments with both our Senators and Congressional Representatives. To facilitate our travel, Susan reluctantly agreed to ride in a wheelchair through the airports both to and from D.C. - i really don't know if i can overstate how reluctantly she made this concession to ME/CFS. She was not experiencing very high energy during that time period and the stress of lobbying Federal Lawmakers was more than daunting - it was crushing, nearly to the point of crippling. While Susan clearly recognized the likely cost to her state of health, her commitment to educating our Lawmakers was greater than the probable consequences. We pressed on.

She had carefully prepared letters for each appointment as well as some information that has been incorporated into this book. The Solve ME organization had also provided a well done packet of statistics that are known to persuade lawmakers - or at least give them cover for spending taxpayer dollars on a little known, poorly understood illness. (There are millions of sufferers in the U.S. alone.) The printed materials we carried with us were hopefully going to be a significant aid in dealing with the very real possibility of cognitive "brain fog" that a day of considerable stress brings. Even when that stress was chosen by you for the best of reasons. Remember, this illness has profound impact on sensory and neurological functioning. It's not as simple as getting really tired. We both knew she was pushing to the edge of collapse. By the end of our third formal lobbying meeting of the day, i had to help Susan physically rise from her chair. Even when exhausted, she had kept on point and acquitted herself beautifully. The Administrative Assistant who had attended that last meeting with our local Congressional Representative, not only recognized her obvious distress but urged us to wait in their office while she got a wheelchair brought up for Susan. No surprise, Susan refused graciously.

Somehow we made it out of the building, with several non-negotiable rest stops. We found a bench near the curb where i nervously propped Susan up in stifling D.C. heat and oppressive humidity. It seemed impossible to get a cab at the end of day rush hour. Finally, i got a cab hailed. Honestly, i'm still not sure how i managed to pour Susan into that cab. She was limp with exhaustion and struggling to breathe. i hated how familiar my fear was. i am not exaggerating or overstating her condition. To this day she has only the vaguest remembrance of that cab ride. i strongly considered having our driver take us to the nearest ER.

A last resort, but one i was aware i might need. Mercifully, the air conditioning in the cab began to work its restorative magic and Susan's breathing slowly improved during the half hour drive through rush hour traffic. We made it back to our affordable but clean Motel. (Rooms at the official event Hotel were much more comfortable and far more expensive. We were there for work, not vacation. Motel it would be.)

The cab let us out in the sizzling parking lot of the Motel with Susan only slightly refreshed. She was able to stand and walk with assistance a few steps at a time. We were then confronted with the outside stairway to our room on the second floor. Twenty some steps that seemed like an obstacle course for elite Ironman/ woman athletes.

Gallantly, and most practically, i offered to carry Susan up those stairs. i was scared enough and pumping enough adrenaline i coulda' done it. Of course, Susan refused, emphatically! No public displays of weakness - she was recovering enough to be a pain. We climbed those stairs in 2 or 3 step increments, resting at least a minute after each exertion. Again, not exaggerating. Upon getting into our affordable room, she dropped on the bed with no attempt to get undressed. i got the room as cool and as dry and her as comfortable as was possible. I turned on T.V. so my close observation of her wouldn't be too obvious. i need not have worried about "hovering" (which Susan really dislikes). Susan had passed out within less than five minutes. Scary times doing good work in D.C. - at least for me.

i was profoundly relieved when she awakened several hours later and actually asked for help getting to the bathroom. An extremely rare ask. The bathroom was less than ten feet from the bed. She was still profoundly weak and cognitively fuzzy, but her breathing was deeper and steadier. Back in bed she was again asleep in minutes and slept through the night. We had known this sort of reaction was beyond possible and had booked an extra day for recovery time after the event. She needed it; more than either of us had imagined. The next day Susan had very little appetite but complied with my insistence that she drink adequate amounts of water. i managed to feed us by gathering provisions from the meager pickings in the Motel lobby vending machines. No room service, no close by restaurants, no elevator left me with a new appreciation of the cost of an affordable alternative Motel.

With very little objection Susan put a wheelchair to good use in navigating our way through the D.C. airport. With extraordinary effort we had both hoped would not be necessary, we made it home. Susan was bedfast for ten days and required assistance to and from the bathroom for the first three of those ten days. She could not have adequately fed herself then. She was effectively home bound for a total of three and a half weeks. This is in no way a "sob story, or poor me tale". This is a report of a silly little "Syndrome". Chronic Fatigue, Yuppie Flu. A Syndrome that can steal your energy so completely you are bed bound. A Syndrome that renders you so tired you literally can not think straight. This is not a complaint. This is a report about a serious condition that is not yet a "Disease". There is also significant physical pain that most patients are given medication to address. i know she has substantial pain and chronic ongoing discomfort but i have never known of Susan to even mention this symptom to a physician. Honestly, i can't remember her ever even complaining of pain. Please recall the biographical information i have shared - another considerable discomfort for Susan. Be very very clear, Susan, like so many other ME/CFS patients, would rather be back at work, and *over* working at that. My point: ME/CFS is real and needs to be respected and have research funded at appropriate levels that are proportional to the severity of the condition, and the real prevalence of its occurrence. It may get ugly. DO NOT GIVE UP!

Over those three and a half weeks, Susan fought back. Recovery in slow motion. Recovery from a kind of fatigue nearly unrecognizably removed from your ordinary garden variety of "tired". Hour by hour, day by day, week by week recovering from participating in an event that would not have been very far removed from the energy demands of any given day of stress in her Area Director position. Recovery from an event she believed was of critical importance. If you have read this and disagree i seriously [well beyond sincerely] suggest you not tell her.

SOME UNSOLICITED ADVICE:

If you are a family member or caregiver with a ME/CFS patient in your life, recognize how serious and life altering this strange stuff that doesn't make you "look sick" truly is. Let them know you believe they are dealing with a major illness. Let them know you are clear they are not faking it or pretending to be sick. Be present with them. DO NOT offer pity. Pity is a Pit that will trap you both.

Do your best to say, "I'm Sorry" as little as possible. (No one close to this misery can resist. Just reset and move on.). DO NOT attempt to "fix it". Don't even think in those terms. Instead find small comforts, pleasant distractions; focus on discovering what soothes and brings even a little relief. Small moments of soothing, distraction, humor and little bits of relief can get woven together to provide significant and meaningful comfort. Educate yourself about both the research and resources meaningful to ME/CFS. Be a focused and relentless advocate. Be willing to do tough things with sometimes difficult people. Focus on small pieces of the big puzzle. And somehow find the presence of mind to allow others to be "right" as long as you get what you want and need for your ME/CFS patient. Be willing to both Ask for help, And Accept help. Build a support network; nurture that network. And take care of yourself - you got folks who need your best. You will never need to be perfect - don't waste precious time and effort on "perfect". Doing your best, day to day, whatever your best is that day will be far more than good enough. Make laughter, fun, and sense of humor a priority. Humor is a lifeline. Being a caregiver is always a dynamic process where the only thing that doesn't change, is the unseen change that's coming next. Expect to make the best you can of each day. Some days will feel lots better than others. Don't worry, it'll change. Be Willing. Be Present.

Believe in Healing: Theirs and Yours.

ONWARD.

And smile like you mean it.

POSTSCRIPT

Update of Current Status

late December 2019 - early January 2020

I am writing this postscript three weeks after the events of the Friday and Saturday i will describe, occurred. Know that Susan had been feeling generally well for the three weeks prior to the weekend on which i'm reporting. She was even physically strong enough and mentally clear enough to drive short distances on several days. The ability to drive has become the Gold Standard of wellness for Susan.

Just after Christmas (2019), our favorite Ohio football team had advanced to the final four in the college playoffs. We are big fans; if you're from Ohio, being a college fan is nearly always more rewarding than being a fan of either of our Pro teams. We were not only excited about The Game but were even more excited about hosting a Game Watching Party for family visiting from Ohio (we are fortunate to be spending the nasty Winter months very near the beach in Florida). The Friday before our scheduled Game Party, we went shopping for supplies in the morning; the early afternoon was then spent in party prep. This is an activity that Susan very much enjoys. i try to stay out of her way and do as i'm told re: cleaning, decorations, and food prep. By now, you may have guessed, Susan has fairly specific plans. Be clear, i am truly happy to receive instruction as long experience has proven that her plans produce swell events, especially parties.

We left several preparation chores go until Saturday morning for a very good reason. A friend we have made here in Florida, a truly accomplished musician/ songwriter/ performer had an early evening gig at a club about 20 minutes from our condo. We are both really big fans and a chance to catch him locally was a real treat - even though it's worth the drive to hear "Boukou Groove" in New Orleans where he often appears. We got to the club early, visited a minute, got great seats and enjoyed two terrific sets. We left after bidding a fond farewell - complete with sweaty hugs (musicians, go figure). We chose to miss what promised to be a "kickin" third set. It was getting tired out and we had a party to stage. We had both enjoyed a larger dose of Fun than ought to be allowed. Well entertained and ready for more, we got to bed around midnight. Very late for Susan.

Susan was noticeably tired the next morning but it was GAME PARTY DAY, and we had seven very welcome guests visiting from back home. We got busy - pretty much all day. Our guests arrived around 5:00 pm (for a 7:00 pm kickoff). Boisterous visitation ensued immediately and the volume level in our condo shot up, only to get significantly louder during the GAME. The final score of the game aside, the party and the visit were more than a success. The "Kids" left around midnight after warm hugs all around. We had no trouble leaving non perishable party debris wait until morning. After tossing spoilables into the refrigerator, we dragged ourselves to bed. Again Big and Welcome Fun - Two Nights in A Row!

Then Sunday morning dawned. We had discussed going to church the day before and i was feeling pretty spry (for an old-ish guy), even with the bitter football loss (in fact, the nasty taste has not yet washed out). Still, i felt refreshed enough to go to church. i had slept and felt generally rested after nearly seven hours of sleep, waking with happy memories of two days of nurturing fun. Susan, not so much.

Susan forced herself to get out of bed and made it to the bathroom with no help. She was profoundly tired. Sleep had not brought any significant refreshment. She awakened more fatigued than when she went to bed. i could hear it in her voice. i could see it in her gait and posture - she was simply too fatigued to stand up straight; let alone move about in her normal smooth gait and impeccable posture. i suggested she simply accept the bill due for two consecutive evenings of fun and head back to bed for a day of clearly needed rest. She, not surprisingly, refused - saying she wanted to sit on the couch for a few minutes before starting to get ready to go to church. (Her "blessing or curse?" persistence on full display - at least to me.) It didn't take a specialist in autoimmune disorders or an expert in sports performance physiology to recognize she was once again struggling with extreme Post Exertion Malaise (again i believe PEM to be a crucial defining characteristic of ME/CFS).

Recall that we had both enjoyed the same social activities. We shared the same sleep schedule. Neither of us had consumed alcohol the previous two days. i got tired too BUT i had recovered, reasonably well for a 72 year old utterly disappointed fan. Susan got tired after nearly identical exertion AND she awakened Sunday radically more tired, weakened, aching, mentally fuzzy, hypersensitive to both light and even moderately loud T.V. volume; and with understandably greater emotional distress than before a night's sleep. While waking up both "sick" and "tired" is all too familiar for people dealing with ME/CFS; waking up this sick and tired was just plain frightening - for both of us.

She couldn't comfortably sit up on our couch. She certainly was not going to church. She did implore me to, "Go ahead and go without me, I'll be fine". As usual, she was concerned and considerate even when in acute distress. (Now somebody else got to be stubborn.) She spent the day in bed; i left the T.V. on, at a low volume, tuned to a channel she normally enjoys - just for distraction if she did awaken. She had no interest in food. This was undeniably a major episode of collapse. She finally felt well enough to sit up in bed for a light snack (i forced on her). She lay back down within 15 minutes and promptly fell asleep again - she slept until 8:45am Monday morning, a very late sleep in for Susan.

While she still felt "totally crappy", a technical medical term, she refused to spend a second day in bed. This was a fight and it was on - bed hair and all. She was determined to answer the bell round after round. She's a Champ, and Champions might get knocked down but they get right back up; and they certainly don't quit. She had set a goal to stay out of bed, even though she was fighting back a migraine (another symptom that has arisen in the past several years - never experienced prior to ME/CFS). She forcefully refused my suggestion to go ahead and take the prescription medication her specialist had written for her. The refusal was even more forceful when i offered the suggestion a second time. i knew better than to make it a third time. Fierce little women can be quite difficult.

Thus, we engaged the most therapeutic strategy available to us. We snuggled on the couch and watched a film festival worth of "B" Christmas movies on Netflix and Amazon Prime; we enjoyed snacks left over from the party and Susan took several unplanned naps. i'm most sincere about our cuddled - mindless "B" Christmas movie film festival viewing. It was soothing. Those times you can't fix it and you can't solve it, learn to reach for simple relief and pleasant distraction and just soothe it. Relief is often enough to get you through rough patches and allow you to regain enough strength to seek some sort of solution. For us Soothing and Relief have become trusted allies. Healers.

Sunset came and we went to bed to continue our festival viewing. Susan was again quickly (30 minutes) asleep. i turned down the volume on the T.V. and watched until sleep found me as well. i was up around 7:00am, fairly normal for me; i was refreshed. Susan again slept until nearly 9:00am, sleeping in for her. She was not yet refreshed by Tuesday morning, but she was a lot further away from despair. Tuesday brought more mediocre Christmas films, but with periodic breaks to check current news developments. She was a little hungry and wanted a cup of coffee. In the afternoon she read a little and started to make some format adjustments to this book; she stopped when another headache threatened to ignite. Again to bed an hour after dark. Again quickly asleep. i was not yet breathing that much sought after "sigh of relief", but i felt optimistic that it was closer - after three days of "holding my breath".

On Wednesday, Susan was awake by 6:00am and wanting to see what was being reported on the morning news shows. Clear signs of recovering. Most encouraging for me, the rasp was gone from her voice. For lunch we had a nice salad and, as usual, she didn't finish all of hers. Good to see another sign of normal. After lunch was the first we dared to utter the dreaded "R" word - RELAPSE. We neither were willing to say it until we felt she had avoided it.

Slowly, but steadily she continued to regain physical strength and cognitive clarity.

Now, three weeks on, Susan continues to gather strength. While she is not yet able to drive again; we are enjoying slow hand in hand walks on the beach. She is caught up on emails and updates on the activities of family members (all family members). She's also paying our bills online, tracking my online medications, and Googling whatever curiosity vexes either of us. We are likely to make it to church this coming Sunday. But no big plans just yet. ME/CFS is a formidable foe. Cautious and expectant optimism is our path of choice. Big platters of Humor, Relief, and Soothing are always on the menu.

Two consecutive days of perfectly reasonable and enjoyable exertion had evoked what seems like a tidal wave of ME/CFS misery and fear. While i can't say either of us expected such a radical consequence, i will freely share we were both all too aware of that unwanted possibility. i've learned that for Susan there will be no other choice than to live brave and invest her "good energy days" in activities that we enjoy. i have also learned that there is no guarantee that taking a preventative "day of rest" will pay off with increased energy on the day you want it. Of course, neither of us are reckless, we plan to rest forward prior to events we know are likely to tax Susan's stamina. An inconvenience that has become a grudging fact of life. A factor Susan never mentions outright - even to family and friends. It's just too damn complicated to quickly explain. For most folks that know her, this will be the first they have heard of the daily challenges of ME/CFS (except, of course, our son Chad who lived it with us at a younger age). Again, this reminder: Pity is not sought, it is of no real use, and it will be summarily rejected.

So we work on balance and conscious appreciation of what's going well. Enjoying our family and friends, learning to be retired together. For me, our hand holding walks on the beach are a most succulent refreshment and source of renewal - she better say the same. There is really nothing better than being madly in love with Susan. And i realize there is very little likelihood of intentional rest in life with Susan. i will simply prepare best as i can to follow her into the next enterprise she dreams up. Yesterday she was talking about she and i collaborating on a family therapy themed book - now there's a major threat to my Netflix watch list.

i hope these recollections have helped you know my WONDER FULL Susan a little better. i also assure you, your ongoing caregiver efforts are essential and well worth any trouble you encounter. It is my sincere hope you find these reflections of some practical use.

Finally, and this time i really mean "finally", Susan is simply my hero.

AND, i really do know how lucky i am.

EPILOGUE

As I bring closure to this book, I struggle with an ending.

Perhaps because writing this book began so many years ago, struggling with my concentration and multiple cognitive limitations that didn't exist prior to Myalgic Encephalomyelitis, made it feel nearly impossible that my end goal would ever be achieved. However, if I hadn't taken the first step of writing that first sentence, that first word, that first foggy ME thought would never have ended in a completed book.

I again encourage you to allow others to help you. This story would not have been told without assistance from my husband, without support from Dr. Meisterman, without the medical knowledge of Dr. Hackshaw, and without the love and caring of my family and friends. Not only do you need to allow others to help you, I learned with much hesitation and difficulty you need to actually ask for help. Sounds easy. Trust me, it's not. A learning lesson for me.

As 2020 arrives next week, it seems a fitting timeframe to bring closure to the writing of this book. As you have previously read, my second bout of this illness began in 2001. I have made gradual improvement, albeit with constant ups and downs as the normal. At times my future thinking has vacillated between being hopeful about a treatment and cure for this frustrating illness, to feeling hopeless about ever having my body return to normal. Thankfully, I have learned to quickly shift my thoughts back to hopeful ones!

Something happened to me mid-March of 2019, nine and a half months ago. I began feeling stronger with improved cognitive processing. I have had no major relapses with only four occurrences of weakened states requiring 24 hour bed rest. Then I was back up and out again. I remain very aware when I am beginning to tire, and I stop myself and rest. I know when to miss activities that I really want to attend or do, to avoid a relapse. I am still unable to drive most days, but I do drive short distances whenever I physically can. So it is not perfect, but it is perfectly wonderful! I have no idea why I improved. Nothing changed in my medications or in my life style. I just improved. I have decided to accept it, and enjoy every day that I can get out of bed and live life as normally as possible. It certainly beats having to transport myself to the bathroom on my heads and knees.

I am blessed, and I pray to the universe for all of us everyday.

APPENDIX

Briefly, I will include one paragraph of the letter my physician, Dr. Benadum, sent to the federal judge prior to my hearing. This is the specific paragraph the judge used in his ruling to grant approval to my disability request. This section was actually typed on my Social Security Disability Insurance Approval Letter.*

THIS IS THE SECTION OF THE LETTER THAT WAS USED IN MY DISABILITY DECISION. IT WAS WRITTEN BY MY PHYSICIAN, DR. BENADUM, TO THE FEDERAL JUDGE AND TO MY ATTORNEY FOR THEIR USE IN MY DETERMINATION HEARING:

(The) claimant is a child and family therapist and used to work 50-60 hours per week in her own private practice. She was also active in her children's school work and managed to run a mile a day. Since the onset of her disease she no longer has the stamina to even work because of constant fatigue and aching joints. She had to close her office and (break) contracts. In addition to private practice she also conducted trainings and seminars as well as lectured after hours at local hospitals for their public and in-house educational programs. She has attempted several times to participate in trainings with her business partner in which he had done all of the preliminary preparation and she would contribute whatever she was able to during the actual presentation. Her last attempt was August 25 and August 26 of 1988 in which she contributed approximately 2 hours each day and at the end of the training she

*In addition to this letter, my physician also attached all my testing, blood levels, medical chart notes, letters for clinical research inclusion, and patient self-charting from my medical records at St. Joseph's Hospital.

had to be carried to the car due to exhaustion and muscle weakness. This was followed by ten days of complete relapse, the first three days being so fatigued that she had to be helped to the bathroom, meals prepared and helped with personal care.

The remaining seven days she was pretty much confined to her bed except for her carrying out her daily living activities. On good days she can vacuum, do laundry and drive approximately two miles to the local mall to walk and just sit and people watch. These activities are accomplished between periods of rest.

There are other days when she goes right back to bed after breakfast. Usually when she pushes herself she relapses into total exhaustion and takes several days to recover. She has been able to do some sewing, beadwork and making jewelry. According to her, she is able to work on this for about 15 minutes before becoming fatigued. After doing minor household chores patient has to lie down due to excessive fatigue (exhibit 25).

SAMPLE LETTER FOR POLITICAL ADVOCACY:

May 15, 2018
The Honorable Senator Rob Portman
Washington D.C.

Dear Senator Portman:

I am writing to introduce myself and my advocacy for Solve ME/CFS (Myalgic Encephalomyelitis/ Chronic Fatigue Syndrome). I have been ill with ME/CFS since 1987, consisting of two separate episodes. The first episode lasting three and a half years, and my second and current episode beginning in May 2001 with no relief for the past seventeen years.

I have written a book about my experience as a patient, filtered through my professional lens as both a psychotherapist and a state level Dept. of Mental Health Administrator. The manuscript is as yet unpublished. I have selected a few chapters (enclosed) for your perusal to assist in understanding this devastating illness. There are an estimated one to two and a half million Americans with this illness, and an estimated eighteen to twenty four million persons worldwide diagnosed, and undiagnosed with ME/CFS.

We are on Capitol Hill today to ask for **your** help. We need someone to care enough to realize we are home in our beds in Zanesville, in our beds across Ohio, in our beds across the United States and in our beds across the globe, unable to plea for help because we are so very ill.

We need help from the NIH and the CDC to show **respect** and give **dignity** to this extremely confusing disease. We need the NIH and CDC to not only recognize it as a real illness, but also to commit sustained dedication to finding the cause and a cure for ME/CFS.

Millions of taxpayer dollars have been spent on futile treatment of this illness because doctors in the United States and abroad have no idea what this illness is, or how to treat it. As you will read in the few chapters I am sharing, you can begin to calculate the dollars that were wasted on just my treatment. Multiply that by one to two and a half million sufferers and you will begin to realize the financial fiasco the NIH and CDC have created by ignoring this very real disease. We desperately need research dollars dedicated to finding the cause, treatment protocol, and hopefully a cure for ME/CFS.

Your help in addressing this health crisis could benefit thousands throughout Ohio and millions across the country, and the globe. I thank you for your time and consideration. I remain your constituent and your responsibility.

Sincerely and Hopefully,
Rebecca Susan Culbertson
Contact Info: xxxxxxxxxx
iPhone: xxxxxxxxxx
Address: xxxxxxxxxx

REFERENCES: RESEARCH

www.solvecfs.org

www.facebook.com/solvemecfsinitiative

www.youtube.com/solvecfs

www.meaction.net

www.youtube.com, The ME Action Network

TED Talks : Jennifer Brea, Posted Jan. 2017, (17 min. 07 sec.) TED Talk, June 2016. #millionsmissing.

http://www.sciencemag.org/news/2015/02/goodbye-chronic-fatigue-syndrome-hello-seid

Open Medicine Foundation www.omf@omf.ngo

Disability application in the United States: Social Security Administration- www.ssa.gov

Television interview on *20/20 ABC News titled, "Is That What's Wrong With Me?"*, moderated by Hugh Downs on the evening of July 31st, 1986. I phoned ABC News and purchased a written copy of that television interview.

Television interview from *Lifetime Cable* that aired on August 28th and 29th, 1988, titled *"Chronic Fatigue Syndrome"*. I obtained a copy of their on-air interview.

"Unrest", A documentary about Jennifer Brea, a Harvard Ph.D. student, who is bedridden by Myalgic Encephalomyelitis / Chronic Fatigue Syndrome. Available on You Tube and Amazon.

Psychoneuroimmunology Research Society www.pnirs.org

http://scopeblog.stanford.edu/2016/08/17/laura-hillenbrand-leaving-frailty-behind/

http://www.kenwilbur.com/writings/pdf/a_sudden_illness.pdf

*Change Your Thoughts - Jennifer Read Hawthorne www.jennifer-hawthorne.com/articles/change_your_thoughts.html

http://gibbsmagazine.com/CryinLaughing.htm

http://en.wikipedia.org/wiki/Golden_Gate_Bridge#Suicides
According to 2005 estimated statistics, by 2012 there would be approximately a total of 1400+ suicide attempts from the Golden Gate Bridge since the recording began in 1937.**

http://www.newyorker.com/archive/2003/10/13/031013fa_fact

http://www.ME-CFS-FM-News@healthrising.org

GLOSSARY

Blood Titre Test - A titer test is a laboratory blood test. It checks for the presence of certain antibodies in the blood stream. Testing involves drawing blood from a patient and checking it in a lab for presence of bacteria or disease. It is often used to see if someone is immune to a certain virus or needs vaccination.

Chronic Fatigue Syndrome - A disease characterized by profound fatigue, sleep abnormalities, pain, and other symptoms that are made worse by exertion.

Diagnostic and Statistical Manual - The Diagnostic and Statistical Manual of Mental Disorders provides clear descriptions of mental health diagnostic categories in order to enable clinicians to diagnosis, study and treat various mental disorders.

efficacious treatment - In medicine, efficacy is the capacity for beneficial change (or therapeutic effect) of a given intervention (for example a drug, medical device, surgical procedure, or a public health intervention).

emotional release - approach to help you release stress, anxiety, fear and other negative emotions by applying a therapeutic process to the concept of an internal memory storage system.

Epstein-Barr Virus - is one of the most common human viruses in the world. It spreads primarily through saliva. EBV can cause infectious mononucleosis, also called mono, and other illnesses.

etiology - a branch of medical science concerned with the causes and origins of diseases.

Fibromyalgia - Fibromyalgia is a disorder characterized by widespread musculoskeletal pain accompanied by fatigue, sleep, memory and mood issues. Researchers believe that fibromyalgia amplifies painful sensations by affecting the way your brain processes pain signals.

Legionnaire's Disease - Legionnaires' disease is a type of pneumonia caused by legionella bacteria. Legionnaires' disease doesn't spread from person to person. Instead, the bacteria spreads through mist, such as from air-conditioning units for large buildings.

Myalgic Encephalomyelitis - Myalgic Encephalomyelitis (ME), commonly known as Chronic Fatigue Syndrome (CFS) or ME/CFS, is a devastating multi-system disease that causes dysfunction of the neurological, immune, endocrine and energy metabolism systems.

negative transformation - The creative endeavor is a way for one to turn a negative experience into a positive one as a means of transformation and growth. Methods may include journaling, music, and emotional release.

paucity - the presence of something only in small or insufficient quantities or amounts; scarcity. "a paucity of information"

Post Exertion Malaise - post-exertion malaise (PEM) - A notable exacerbation of symptoms brought on by small physical or cognitive exertions. PEM can last for days or weeks. Symptoms can include cognitive impairments, muscle pain (myalgia), trouble remaining upright (orthostatic intolerance), sleep abnormalities, and gastro-intestinal impairments, among others.

primary care physician - is a doctor for treating your medical health-care. I use my PCP as a coordinating physician with my ME/CFS specialist, but you may use your PCP for both medical care and ME/CFS care if they are qualified and willing. In my own experience I have found it better to separate the PCP care from the ME/CFS Specialist care for reasons of medical fatigue and lack of ME/CFS knowledge.

psychoneuroimmunology - Psychoneuroimmunology (PNI), also referred to as psychoendoneuroimmunology (PENI) or psychoneuroendocrinoimmunology (PNEI), is the study of the interaction between psychological processes and the nervous and immune systems of the human body.

suicidal ideation - Suicidal thoughts, or suicidal ideation, means thinking about or planning suicide.Thoughts can range from a detailed plan to a fleeting consideration. It does not include the final act of suicide.

symptomatological treatments - Treatments that address symptoms.

ACRONYM IDENTIFICATION

AAAS   American Association for the Advancement of Science

CDC   Center for Disease Control

CFS   Chronic Fatigue Syndrome

DSM   Diagnostic and Statistical Manual

IOM   Institute Of Medicine

ME   Myalgic Encephalomyelitis

MPF   Medical Provider Fatigue

PEM   Post Exertion Malaise

PCP   Primary Care Physician

PNI   Psychoneuroimmunology

SEID   Symptomatological Exertion Intolerance Disease

SSA   Social Security Administration

SSDI   Social Security Disability Insurance

BIBLIOGRAPHY

Osler's Web, by Hillary Johnson, Crown Publishers, Inc., New York, 1996. ISBN 0-517-70353-X.

The Biology of Belief, by Dr. Bruce Lipton, Mountain of Love/Elite Books, 2005. ISBN 0975991477.

The Diagnostic and Statistical Manual of Mental Disorders : DSM-5, - 5th edition. American Psychiatric Association Publishing, 800 Maine Avenue SW, Suite 900, Washington, DC 20024-2812. ISBN 978-0-89042-554-1 (Hardcover) 5th printing, January 2019.

See Reference : Research Section of this book.

ACKNOWLEDGMENTS

I offer my sincere thanks for the generous assistance of my first readers, Cheryl Wells, LMT, CHt; Michael McVicker, OCPSII; and Dr. Cherla Meisterman, PhD, LISW whose comments and questions were insightful and helpful. I am indebted to my family who have supported me in the past, and to this present day. My lovely parents, Chet & June Culbertson, now deceased, carried soup to my home and cared for me with never a moment of questioning my illness. My sister and her husband, Sharon and Larry Wisecarver who came to my aid whenever I needed medical support and drove me to appointments when I couldn't drive myself. My Auntie Diane Harsh and Uncle William Fortner for their moral support and caring phone calls.

I am overwhelmed and indebted to my medical team, Dr. Ismet Ozkazanc, Dr. Cherla Meisterman, Dr. Connie Jenkins, and Dr. Kevin Hackshaw; and my former team members, Dr. Timothy Benadum and Dr. Maria Jamiolkowski, for their professional excellence and unbelievable empathy shown to me over the months and years of dealing with this confusing illness.

Special thanks and gratitude goes to Dr. Meisterman for her support through my second episode of ME/CFS, and assisting me through my darkest days of grief and loss of my professional self. She encouraged my work on this book and patiently saw me through setbacks and times of relapse. Dr. Meisterman also gave welcome support to my husband as we traveled together through this frustrating confusing illness.

Dr. Kevin Hackshaw, (Kevin V. Hackshaw, M.D. Director of Fibromyalgia Specialty Clinics, Program Director, Rheumatology, The Ohio State University, Columbus, Ohio, Division of Immunology/ Rheumatology), saved me multiple times on my confusing journey through ME/CFS Land. Dr. Hackshaw has been there for me at my most seriously ill times during my second episode. He solved mysteries for me at the conclusion of hospitalizations resulting in zero answers from multiple inpatient care doctors; and he prevented unnecessary hospitalizations with swift, decisive actions formulated from his vast knowledge of how to diagnose and treat ME/CFS symptoms. I will never allow myself to be hospitalized or treated for ME/CFS symptoms without consulting Dr. Hackshaw for his opinion prior to any future actions on my behalf. I trust him literally with my life. Thank you, Dr. Hackshaw, for bringing such comfort and security to my life! I have no way of ever repaying you - I say simply, "Thank you"!

My never ending support goes out to every person worldwide suffering, with or without a diagnosis of Myalgic Encephalomyelitis. I pray everyday for a cure for all of us. I thankfully acknowledge the current dedicated and tireless researchers. In particular, Dr. Ronald W. Davis of the Open Medicine Foundation (omf.ngo) and Dr. Nancy G. Klimas, M.D. of Nova Southeastern University, who are seeking that cure for all ME sufferers.

I sincerely thank my fellow colleagues at the Ohio Dept. of Mental Health in Columbus, Ohio, who still stun me by having gifted their precious vacation and sick time when I had nothing left to carry me through to disability. Who does that? Only really good people. And you all did it anonymously! Who does *that*? Really, *really* good people. You brought me to tears. Thank you. I will carry your goodness with me forever. Thank you to my Administrative Supervisor, Judy Wood, LISW, and Director Dr. Mike Hogan who held my position open for months, allowing me time without pressure to attempt to return to my professional role. If I could have, I would have. I truly loved my world of mental health.

I have been richly rewarded with four grandchildren, Allen, Kelsey, Siena and Madelyne, whom have all given me more hugs, laughs and sticky kisses than one could ever count. And now my little great grandson, Archer, who has taken over the role of joy maker. I remain in love with all of you.

Most of all, I thank my husband, Michael, my sons, Jon and Chad, and my daughter-in-laws, Stef and Michelle for their unconditional love and unwavering support throughout not only the writing of this book, but also through the years of fighting this unrelenting illness with it's minuscule progress, followed by it's major setbacks. Frustrations galore, always met with fierce family strength that held me above the devastating attacks. Fierce family strength. Thank you with my whole heart.

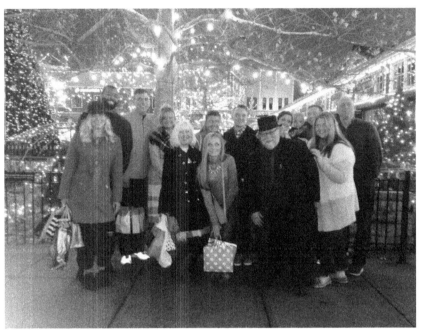

❤*Our Family: Kelsey, Charles, Jon, Stef, Susan, Madelyne, Siena, Parker, Michael, Alison, Archer, Allen, Michelle, and Chad.* ❤

ABOUT THE AUTHOR

Rebecca Susan Culbertson, MSW, LISW-S, is a Child & Family Therapist, and a first time author. She graduated from Ohio University with a degree in Education, and from the University of Denver with a Master's Degree in Clinal Social Work, emphasis on Child & Family Therapy. Rebecca was fortunate to have received monthly supervision sessions for her clinical family therapy work with Dr. Carl Whitaker, until the time of his death in 1995. Rebecca has taught at Universities in both Colorado and Ohio. She has provided psychotherapy services both in the public and private sectors. Her final professional service was in a governor-appointed position as an Area Director of Mental Health for Southeastern Ohio. Rebecca was first diagnosed with ME/CFS (Myalgic Encephalomyelitis) in 1987, and continues her struggle to this day. She currently lives with her husband in Ohio, and is planning retirement in Destin, Florida.

CPSIA information can be obtained
at www.ICGtesting.com
Printed in the USA
FSHW021956090821
83949FS